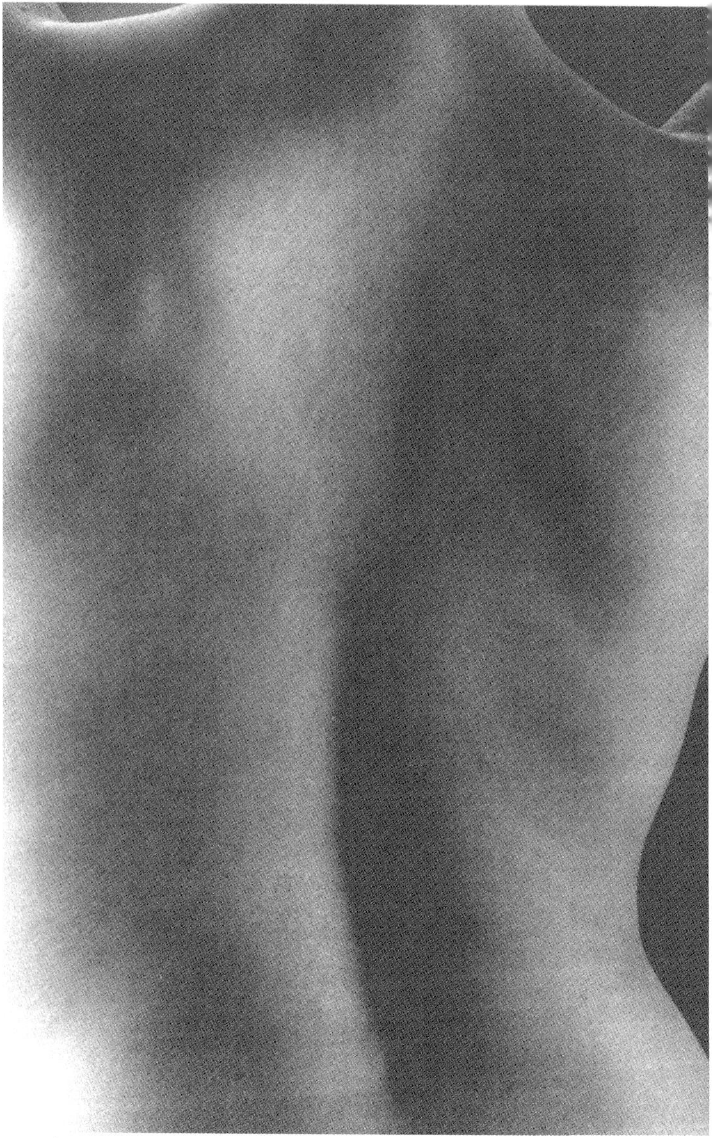

Help Yourself to Health

Back Pain

Practical ways to restore health using complementary medicine

Prof. Edzard Ernst
MD, Ph.D., FRCP (Edin)

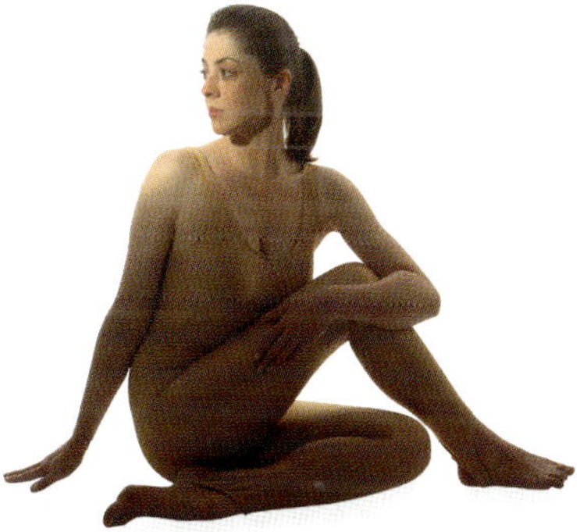

A Godsfield Book

This edition published in Great Britain in 1999
by Godsfield Press Ltd, a division of
David and Charles Ltd, Laurel House, Station Approach
Alresford, Hants, SO24 9JH, U.K.

10 9 8 7 6 5 4 3 2 1

Designed by the
Bridgewater Book Company

Printed and bound in Hong Kong

ISBN 1-899434-68-2

CONTENTS

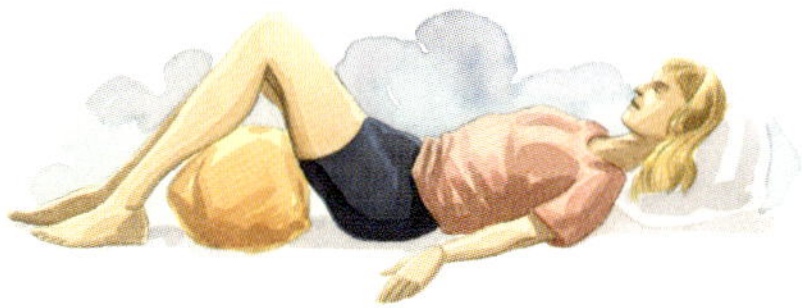

INTRODUCTION

BACK PAIN IS SO COMMON *that some experts now say that it is the norm. In other words, it is not the person with back problems who is remarkable, but the person who is entirely free of them. Indeed, 80 to 90 percent of us will suffer from back trouble at least once in our lifetime: it is the second most frequent complaint after the common cold.*

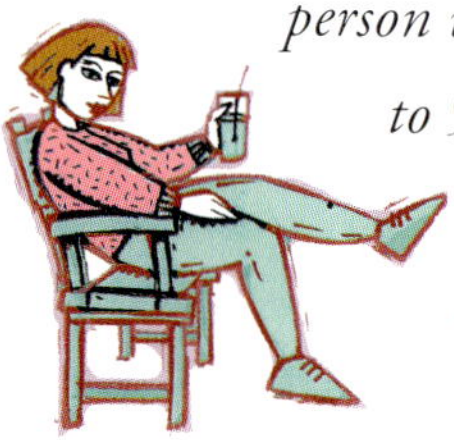

ABOVE *It's easy to adopt a bad posture without thinking.*

Because there is no easy and absolute cure for back pain, general physicians are often at a loss to know how to deal with it. Today back pain is the most common reason for people to consult complementary practitioners.

Complementary (sometimes still wrongly called "alternative") medicine has become enormously popular over the last twenty years. About a third of Americans and a quarter of Britons have tried at least one complementary therapy during the last year.

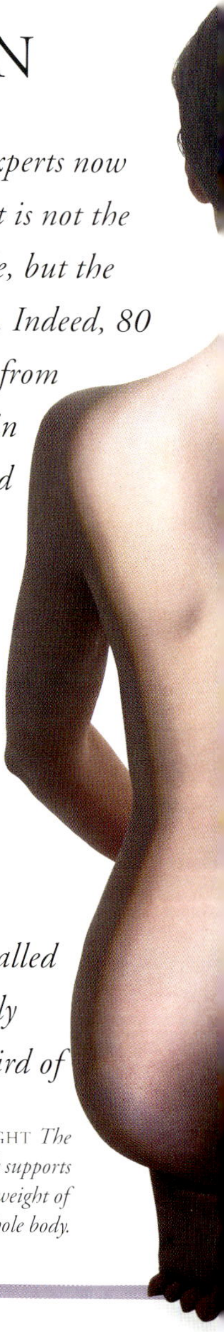

RIGHT *The back supports the weight of the whole body.*

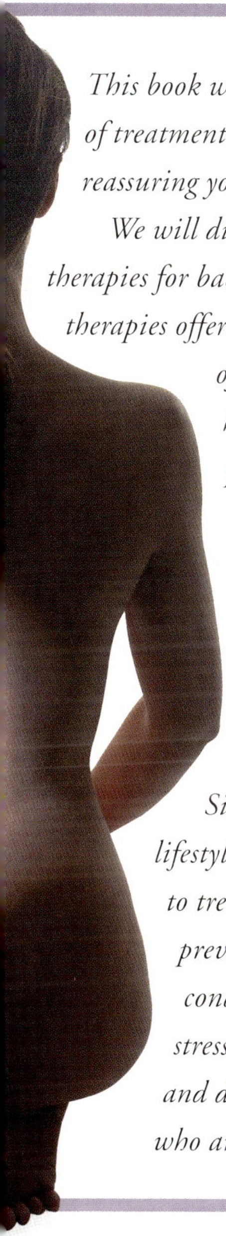

This book will take you step by step through the jungle of treatment options. It is a practical guide, aimed at reassuring you and helping you to cope.

We will discuss the most promising complementary therapies for back pain, and briefly look at relevant therapies offered by mainstream medicine. The best way of dealing with back pain is to prevent it happening in the first place. The book will provide you with useful tips about what to do, and what to avoid, including a separate chapter on back pain and sport. Simple changes in lifestyle may go a long way to treating and helping to prevent an annoying condition that causes stress, discomfort, pain, and disability for those who are affected.

COMPLEMENTARY THERAPIES

- Manipulation
- Acupuncture
- Massage
- Alexander Technique
- Healing
- Herbalism
- Homeopathy
- Reflexology
- Yoga

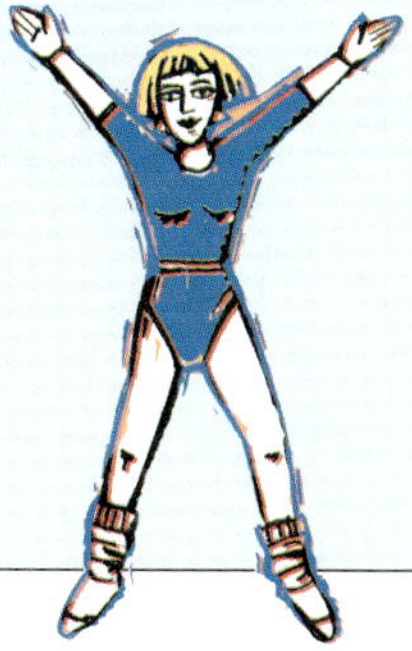

WHAT IS BACK PAIN?

Back pain comes in many guises. The pain can be constant, or present only on certain occasions (such as when standing or walking), or it may be totally unpredictable.

The pain may be confined to the back, but it can also radiate into the buttocks or into the leg. The sensation can be anything from a deep aching pain to a sharp stabbing pain, a diffuse burning pain, or a distinct nerve pain.

BELOW *Back pain takes many forms, even when it is non-specific.*

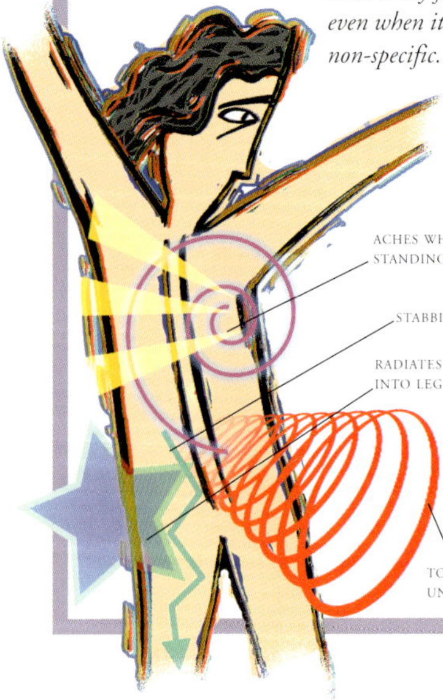

THE MANY CAUSES OF BACK PAIN

Back pain, like any other pain, is certainly not a disease. It is a symptom. This means that we have to consider the cause of the symptom. And back pain can have many causes.

The list of causes may make you shudder. It is obvious that some of these are very serious conditions. But in more than 90 percent of all cases, back pain is not caused by one of these illnesses. Unable to directly attribute the cause of the pain, a physician is likely to refer to your condition as either:

- *"Non-specific" back pain.*
- *"Idiopathic" back pain.*
- *"Mechanical" back pain.*

POSSIBLE SPECIFIC CAUSES OF BACK PAIN

Difference in leg length

Fractures of the vertebrae

Hypermobility of the spine or a segment of the spine

Infections of or around the spine

Osteoporosis

Paget's disease

Psychogenic problems

Referred pain from inner organs

Rheumatic diseases

Scoliosis (abnormal twisting of the spine)

Sickle cell disease

Slipped disk

Spinal stenosis (a narrowing of the inner lumen of the spinal canal)

Spondylolisthesis (a congenital abnormality of the bony structures of the spine)

Tumors

CANCER

The most threatening cause of back pain is cancer, although this is very rare. The factors listed below are indicators that should alert you and your physician to the possibility of cancer pain which is masquerading as back pain. If you notice any of these signs, you must discuss them with your physician, who can then investigate further to rule out cancer.

- ☐ Absence of most typical features of "normal" back pain.
- ☐ Constant pain independent of movement or posture.
- ☐ Atypical location of pain.
- ☐ Bone pain also elsewhere in the body.
- ☐ Symptoms other than pain.

NON-SPECIFIC BACK PAIN

A specific cause for back pain exists in only 10 percent of cases, and only a small proportion of these will be serious. Non-specific back pain makes up the majority of cases. Here are some of the characteristics that are likely indicators of this most common category of back pain:

1. *Discomfort across the lower back, or located centrally over your lower spine.*
2. *Pain radiating into the buttocks or legs.*
3. *Recurring episodes of similar back pain in the past.*
4. *Early-morning stiffness.*
5. *Back pain is eased by moving yourself about.*
6. *Pain aggravated by sitting or remaining in one position for some time.*

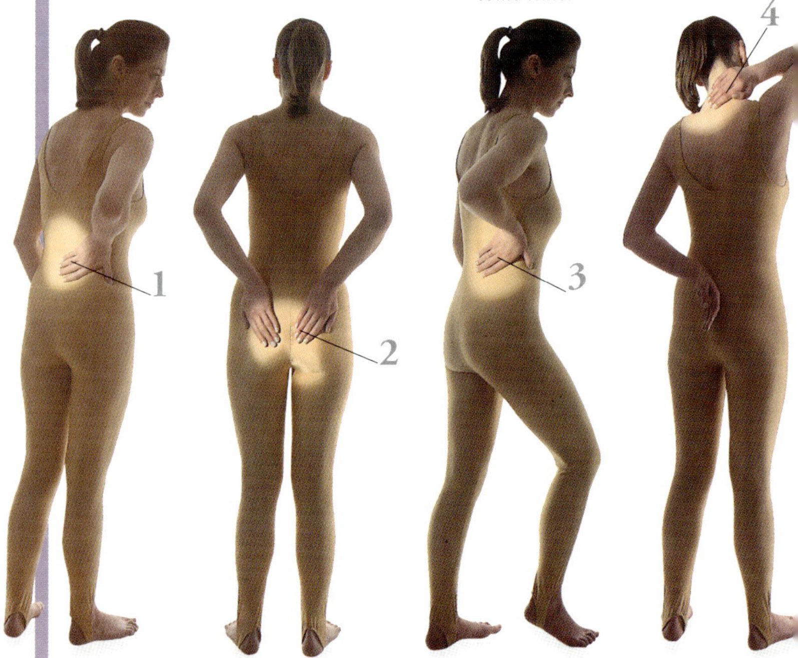

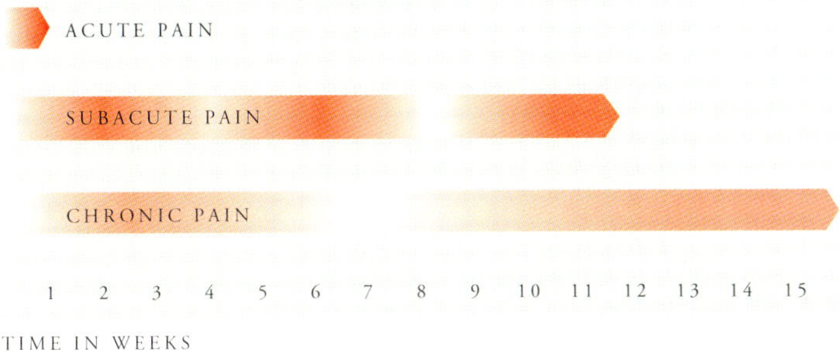

ABOVE *Non-specific pain is described according to duration.*

PAIN CATEGORIES

Even non-specific ("normal") back pain, can be subdivided into a number of further categories. Here are some of them:

- ✧ Acute back pain (lasting up to seven days).
- ✧ Subacute back pain (lasting more or less constantly for a period of up to three months).
- ✧ Chronic back pain (lasting longer than three months without major pain-free periods).
- ✧ Intractable pain (chronic pain that cannot be reduced by any of the non-surgical treatment options).

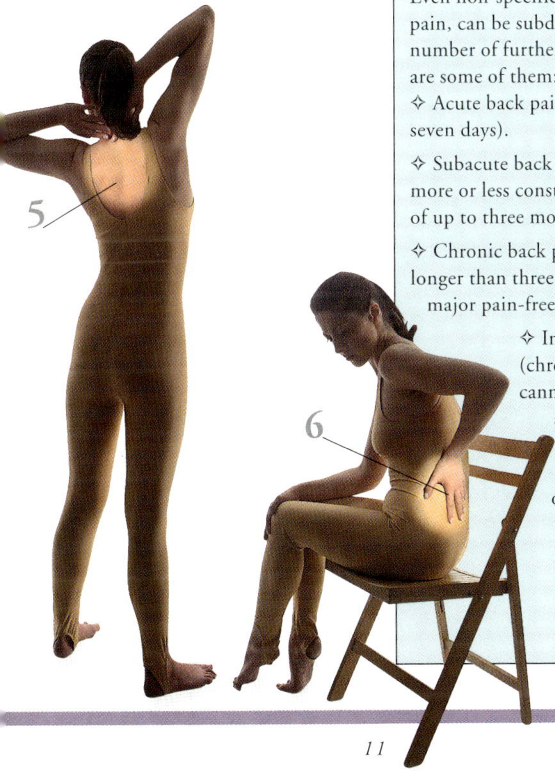

RECOVERY

So let's assume that your physician has examined you and assured you that your pain is of the "normal," non-specific type. What is likely to happen to you?

About 90 percent of sufferers recover from their pain, the vast majority within a week or so. In many cases, however, the pain can recur at a later stage. About 10 percent of sufferers will go on to have chronic back pain. Only 1 percent of sufferers will be severely disabled through their back pain.

OUTLOOK

This means that the prognosis for back pain is extremely good. The important thing is to accept that an episode of back pain is not at all unusual, and to do everything possible to prevent it from becoming chronic. Pay attention to your posture, sit on supportive chairs, sleep on a firm mattress, and take care when lifting. Lose weight if you are overweight, and begin a program of suitable regular exercise.

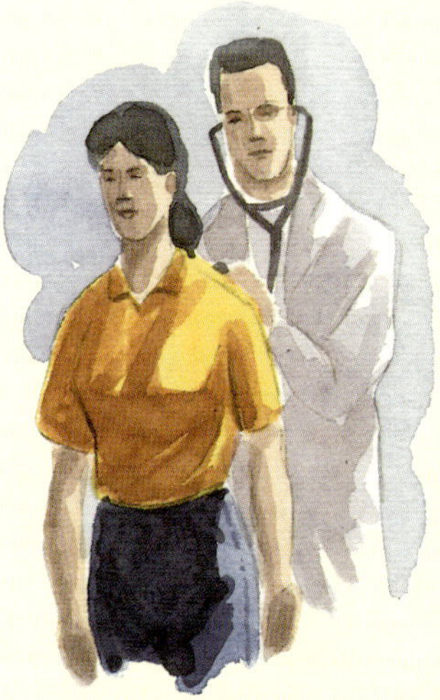

ABOVE *A physician will do a thorough physical examination.*

SEEING A PHYSICIAN

If your back pain gets worse, consult your physician. (Or if you experience any of the following symptoms: weakness, numbness or tingling in the legs, difficulty in passing urine or feces.) Obviously, if the back pain is the result of a serious injury or accident, do not move the patient and call an ambulance or physician immediately for expert treatment.

RECURRENT BACK PAIN

When the pain starts, take painkillers and rest up for a couple of days. Heat may help to relax muscle spasm: sit or lie with a suitably protected heating pad against the painful area. When you are fully mobile again, start doing gentle exercises to build up the muscles of the spine, and help prevent future episodes of pain. Ask your physician for a list of appropriate exercises, or consult a physiotherapist.

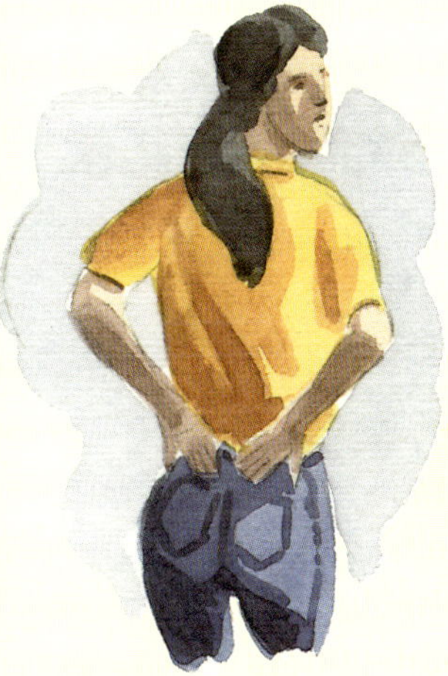

ABOVE *Unfortunately 10 percent go on to chronic back pain.*

SUMMARY

Back pain is extremely frequent; nearly everyone suffers from it at some stage.

✧

Back pain must therefore be considered almost as "normal."

✧

Only in very rare cases is back pain caused by a serious disease. If there are any signs that make you suspect this, discuss your worries with your physician.

✧

The vast majority of cases have no specific causes; they are therefore called "non-specific" back pain. Non-specific back pain is usually nothing to worry about.

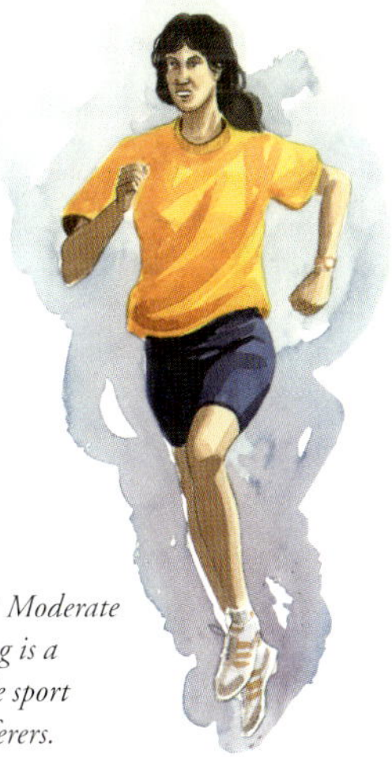

RIGHT *Moderate running is a suitable sport for sufferers.*

STRUCTURE AND FUNCTION OF THE BACK

The spine has complex functions which require a specialized structure. Basically, the spine and its surrounding tissues serve to protect, to support, and to facilitate motion.

THE SPINAL CORD

All the sensations from the periphery of the body are transmitted as nerve signals to the "central computer," the brain. The brain controls many body functions and sends its commands, via the nerves, back to the body. Most of these ascending and descending signals are carried in the spinal cord.

The brain sends signals to the body through the nervous system, which are carried in the spinal cord.

At the spaces between the vertebrae, the spinal cord branches into nerve roots.

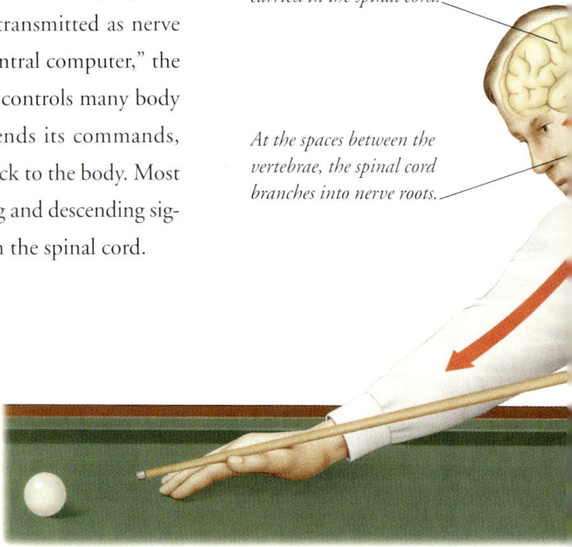

RIGHT *The spinal cord is carried in the spinal column, where it is protected by bone.*

The spinal cord is like a big cable connecting the central nervous system with the periphery. It is therefore a most delicate structure, as delicate as the brain itself. Just as the brain is protected from external injury by the skull, the spinal cord is protected by the bony structures of the spinal column. From the point where the spinal cord leaves the skull, and all the way down to the tail bone, it is surrounded by a strong shield called the spinal column.

THE SPINAL COLUMN

The spinal column consists of twenty-four bones called vertebrae. It can be subdivided into several sections: the cervical spine (neck), the thoracic spine (chest), and the lumbar spine (lower back). All vertebrae have a similar structure. They form a hollow canal in which the spinal cord lies. In the gaps between each vertebra run the nerves transmitting information to and from the spinal cord.

BODYGUARD

This unique structure thus provides an ideal protection for the functionally highly specialized and mechanically vulnerable spinal cord. This protection is essential, because even a slight injury to the cord causes utter chaos for the nervous system, possibly even total paralysis or death.

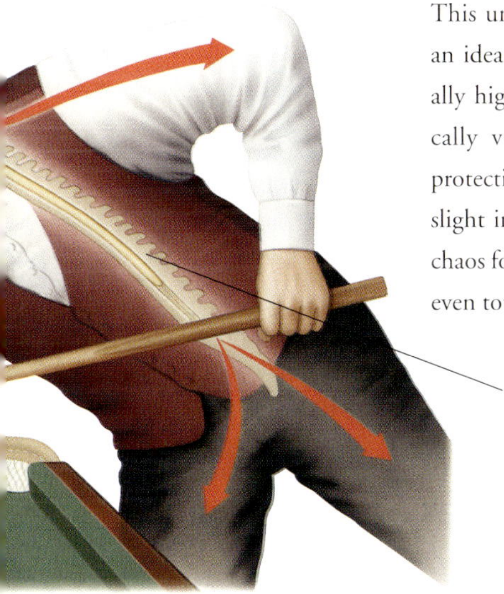

The spinal cord ends at the top of the lumbar vertebrae, where it branches off into many nerve roots which carry on downwards through the spinal canal.

THE SPINE AS A MECHANICAL SUPPORT

The bones of the spine, the vertebrae, form the major pillar of our body. The vertebrae are divided into five sections, depending on where they are in the spine: cervical (neck), thoracic (chest), lumbar (abdomen), sacral (connects the spine to the pelvis), and caudal (the tailbone).

Most other bones of the body are hinged on the spinal pillar. The head rests on the cervical spine, the arms are suspended from the thoracic spine with a complex system of interconnections, the ribs are joined to the thoracic spine, and the legs are attached via the pelvis and the tail bone to the lumbar spine. The spine therefore has to be a solid and durable supporting structure.

BUILDING A SOLID STRUCTURE

Because the cervical spine merely carries the weight of the head, its vertebrae are comparatively delicate. Further down the body, vertebrae become more robust in order to carry more weight.

THE INTERLOCKING BUILDING BLOCKS OF THE SPINE

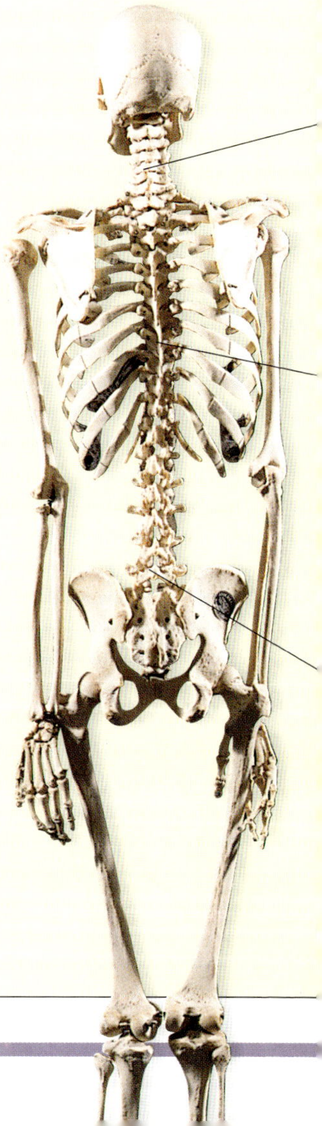

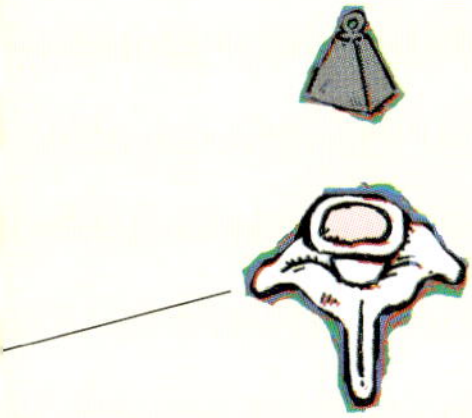

The cervical spine has to carry the weight of the head. Its seven vertebrae are relatively delicate.

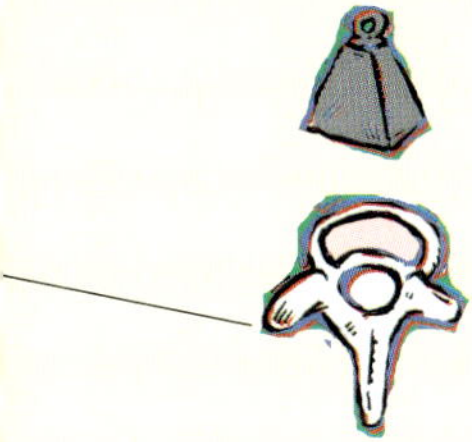

The twelve thoracic vertebrae are bigger, and must support the weight of the arms and ribs.

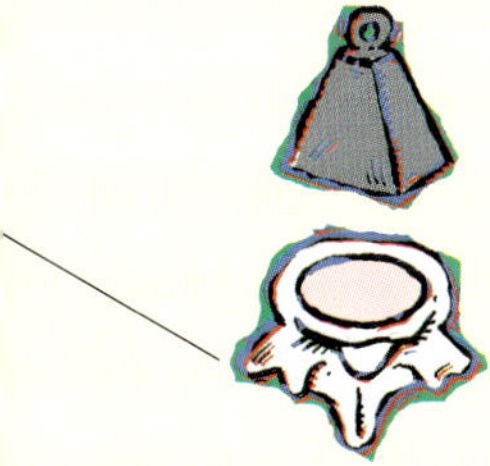

The five lumbar vertebrae are the largest in the spine, as they have to carry the most weight.

Between the vertebrae are the intervertebral disks – cushioning tissue with a gelatine-like center (nucleus pulposus), and a tight and tough crisscross fibrous structure surrounding it (annulus fibrosus). The intervertebral disks have to endure enormous strains, so the annulus fibrosus has to be extremely strong and resilient. For extra strength, the whole assembly is covered by several layers of musculature. This powerful combination is essential for the spine to function as the central pillar of the body. The lumbar spine's ability to withstand compression decreases with age.

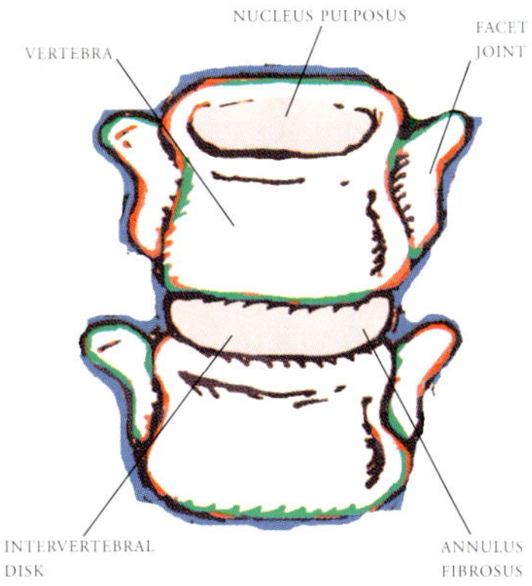

ABOVE *Intervertebral disks between the vertebrae act as shock absorbers.*

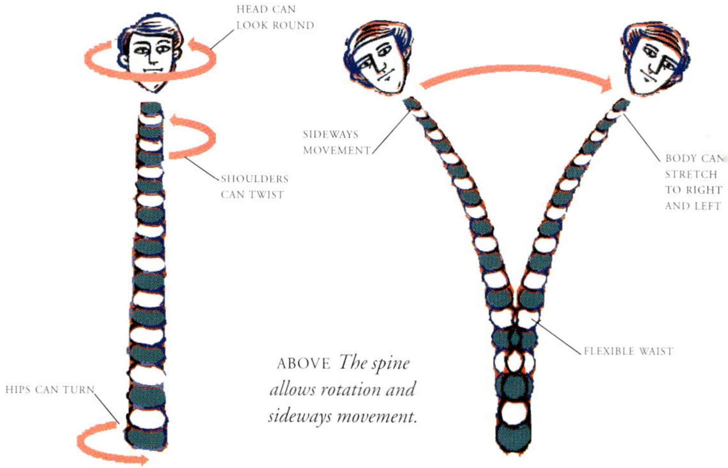

ABOVE *The spine allows rotation and sideways movement.*

THE SPINE AS A FACILITATOR OF MOVEMENTS

If the spine were a rigid tube, it would be strong, but movement would be critically inhibited. But the spine is far from being rigid. It can move sideways in both directions, it can tilt forward and, to a lesser degree, backward, and it can rotate. Different spinal segments have different tasks in terms of contributing to this overall mobility. The cervical spine rotates best, enabling us to look to the left and right. The lumbar spine can tilt forward, so that we can bend our body when we need to.

The remarkable degree of mobility is achieved mainly through small joints that link the vertebral arches. The exact position of these joints varies between spinal segments. It determines the type of movement possible in each motion segment.

Spinal mobility is further enhanced by the elasticity of the intervertebral disks. These act like shock absorbers, because they are filled with fluid. However, the fluid content reduces with age, making us more vulnerable to injury.

RIGHT *Forward and backward flexibility permits bending.*

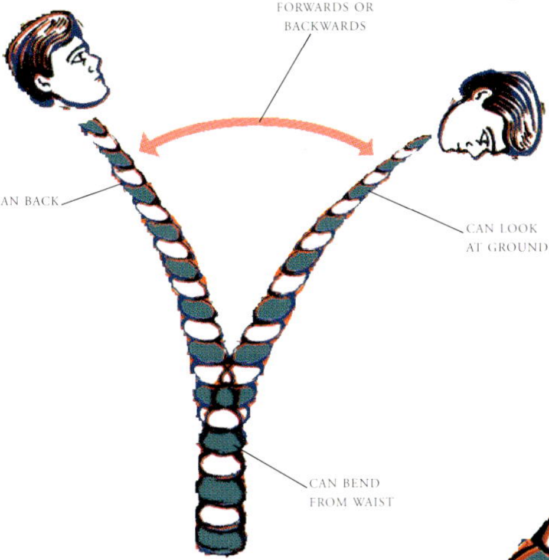

FLEXIBILITY

The ligaments tying up the vertebrae run in such a way that they do not entirely inhibit movement between the motion segments.

While the mobility of each single motion segment is rather small, the spinal column as a whole is very mobile. This effect is achieved because the small movements of each segment add up to an overall mobility of the spine. Thus only a few degrees in one segment mean ninety degrees or more across all twenty-four vertebrae, enabling us to touch our toes.

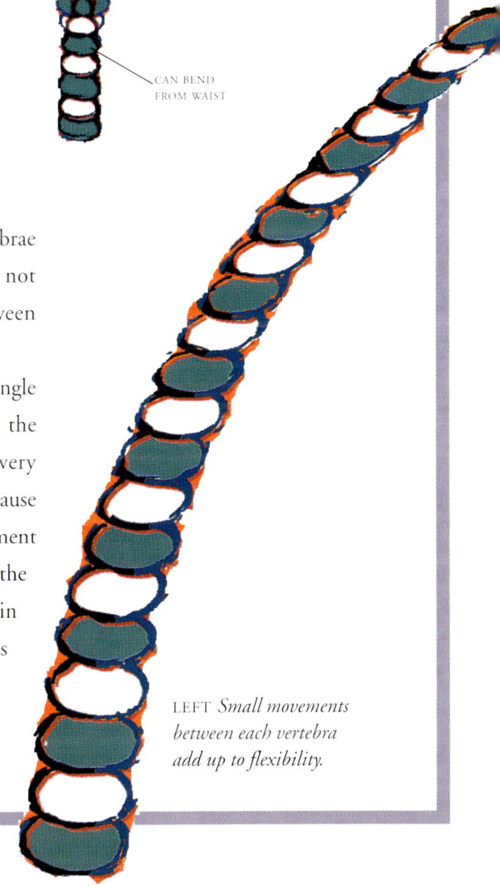

LEFT *Small movements between each vertebra add up to flexibility.*

THE BACK AND THE PSYCHE

There is a close relationship between the mind and the body in general, as well as the mind and the back in particular. Psychological factors may strongly influence the course of back pain – its chronicity, the patient's ability to cope, and the rate of recurrence.

Research shows that factors such as anxiety, mental stress, dissatisfaction with work and monotony of work are associated with higher frequency and severity of back pain. The interaction of these factors can be quite complex. We need to understand them better in order to define their role and improve the treatment and prevention of back pain.

When back pain lasts for months, it is often advisable to see a psychologist, to sort out whether there is a psychological problem that is aggravating the situation. Even if this is not the case, the consultation may lead to better ways of coping.

THE FEAR FACTOR

Fear may be a further important factor in aggravating or prolonging pain. Back pain patients may be frightened that:

Painkillers have side-effects or cause dependency

✧

Leading an active life causes pain or damage to the back

✧

Back pain is caused by a serious disease

✧

Back pain negatively impacts on their life (e.g. loss of earnings)

If you are frightened, discuss your worries with your physician or therapist. Almost invariably, your fears will be ill-founded.

Nowadays, multidisciplinary teams treating chronic back problems include psychologists, with considerable success.

Any long-lasting illness, particularly if painful, will have psychological effects on the sufferer, their family, and colleagues. In some cases, the behavior or even the personality of the sufferer may change. Changes like this are usually a bad sign. It is mandatory that, in such situations, professional help is sought from an experienced psychologist.

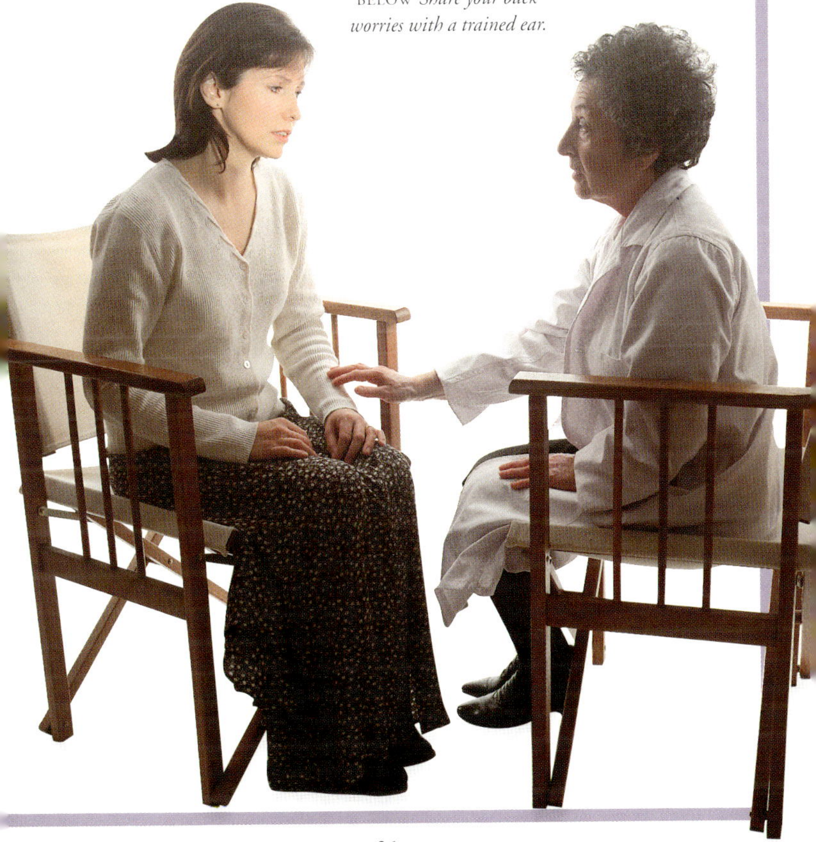

BELOW *Share your back worries with a trained ear.*

CONVENTIONAL TREATMENTS

This book is not about conventional treatments for back pain. It is, however, necessary to briefly mention the options used in mainstream medicine to treat back pain. As a back pain sufferer, you should know about all treatment options.

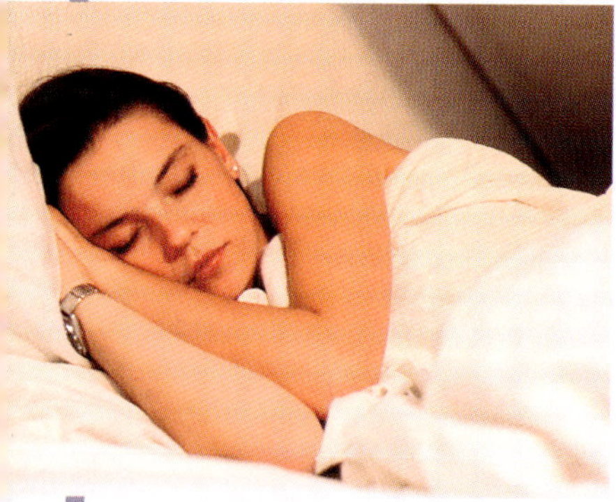

ABOVE *Not the best position for sleeping in during recovery.*

BED REST

Resort to bed rest only when it is unavoidable (for severe pain), and only for a short time. Prolonged bed rest is strongly counterproductive. While in bed, the best position to adopt is usually on your back with a large object under your knees, so that your thighs are raised almost vertically.

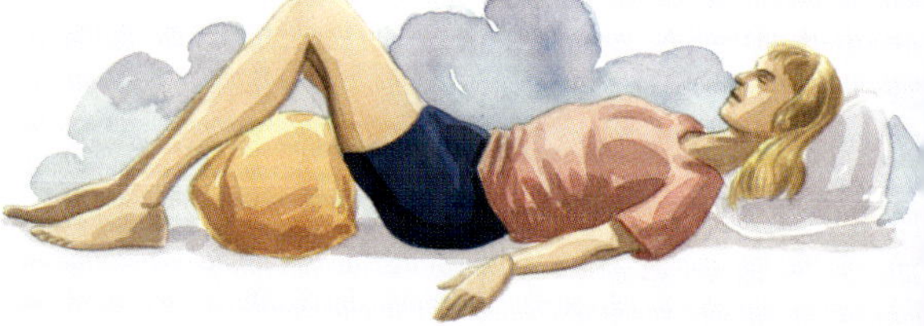

RIGHT *This is better: lie flat with your knees raised.*

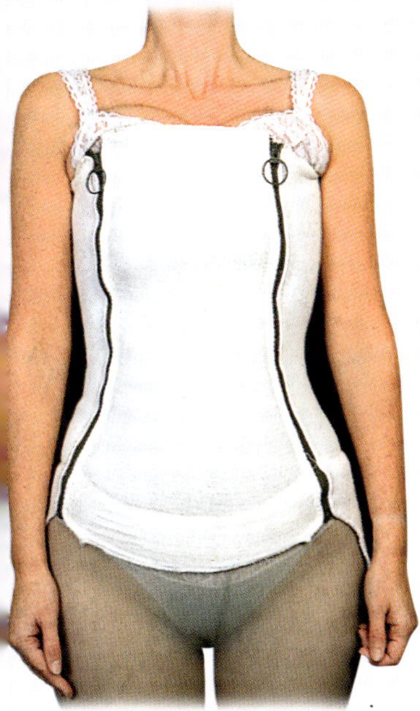

ABOVE *An orthopedic corset may be worn for damaged spinal disks.*

SPINAL SUPPORTS

A number of devices, such as corsets and braces, support your back and immobilize it. This may alleviate the pain, yet it is counterproductive in the long run. Therefore, use only in extreme cases, and if possible not as a long-term solution.

PAINKILLERS

Painkillers can be very helpful, making life bearable during a (short) time of intense pain. But do not use drugs as a long-term solution for back pain. More than half of all back pain patients who see a physician receive prescriptions for "nonsteroidal anti-inflammatory drugs,"and these drugs are burdened with the risk of serious side-effects. One of the best drugs to start with is tylenol.

RIGHT *Painkillers have their place in pain management.*

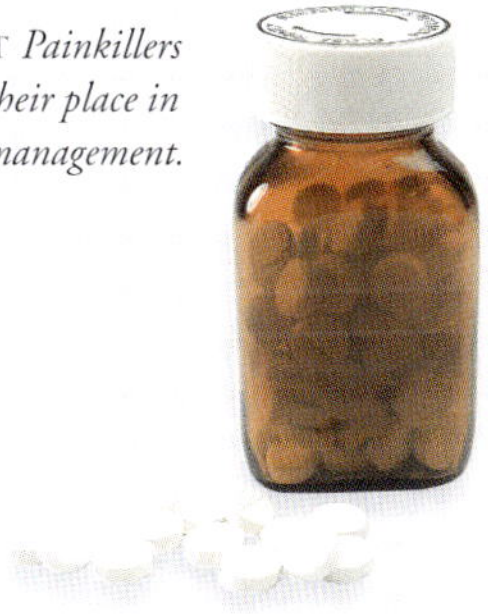

MUSCLE RELAXANTS

These drugs can be helpful for a short while. They reduce muscular tension in the back and therefore relieve pain. Again, do not use drugs for prolonged periods.

TRACTION

Several devices exist to exert a pull on your spine along its longitudinal axis. The idea is to release pressure on trapped nerves. Traction is usually, however, not very helpful. If it is not applied properly, it can even be positively dangerous.

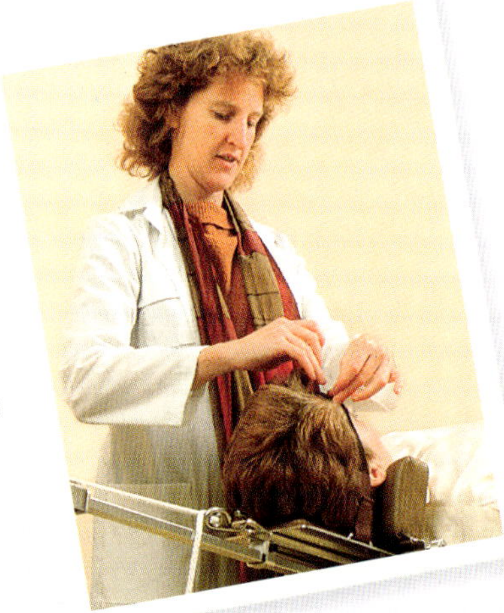

RIGHT *A physiotherapist secures a neck brace on a patient, before she undergoes traction.*

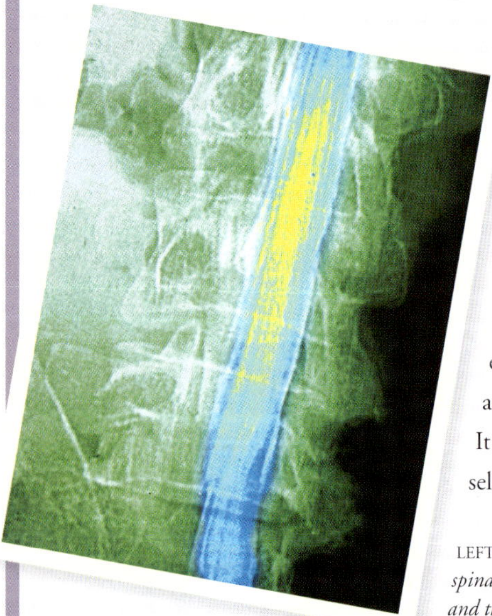

SPINAL CORD STIMULATION

This method can be effective in chronic cases of otherwise intractable back pain. It includes the implantation of electrodes near the spinal cord and therefore carries certain risks. It should only be used in carefully selected cases.

LEFT *A side view of the spinal cord (blue/yellow) and the vertebrae (white).*

SURGERY

There are various operations which, depending on the exact anatomical situation, may be advocated. Generally speaking, surgery for back pain is employed far too often. It should be reserved for desperate cases. Every surgical procedure is burdened with a mostly small, but measurable risk. Many patients who have had surgery nontheless do go on to have further back problems.

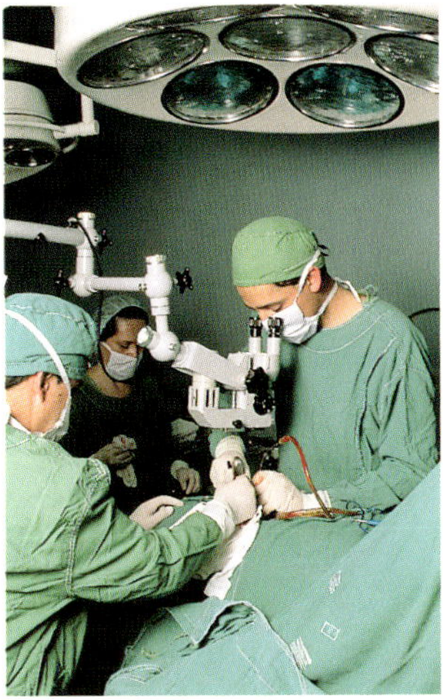

ABOVE *Surgery should be a last resort for serious cases.*

IS IT NECESSARY?

On the other hand, studies show that many patients who were advised to have surgery, but in the end did not, recovered just as quickly as those patients who did undergo surgery. Today, some prominent orthopedic surgeons are therefore highly critical about back surgery. Some go as far as stating that the biggest advance in the successful treatment of back pain would be if surgeons stopped operating on those patients who are not clear cases for surgery.

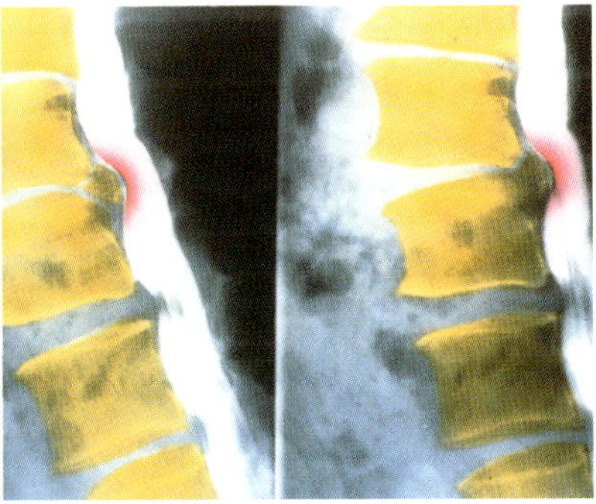

LEFT *A slipped disk which is compressing the spinal cord, causing pain.*

TENS

The abbreviation "TENS" stands for "transcutaneous electrical nerve stimulation." Many experts would say that this is a conventional form of treatment. But as TENS is often used by complementary practitioners, it makes sense to discuss it here.

THE CONCEPT

TENS is a modern development. In principle, it works through electric impulses which are generated by a small, battery-powered electronic device. Two cables are attached to the skin by electrodes, usually in the region of the pain. The type (strength and frequency) of these impulses can be varied. They can be so small that they are not noticed by the patient, or they can be upgraded until a slight sensation is felt.

The electrical impulses stimulate nerve fibers and are transmitted towards the brain. It is thought that, on their way, they induce complex changes at nerve interconnections. This, in turn, would alter the way these nerves conduct pain signals to the brain. It is hoped that, with the right TENS impulse, pain conduction is partly inhibited and therefore less pain is felt.

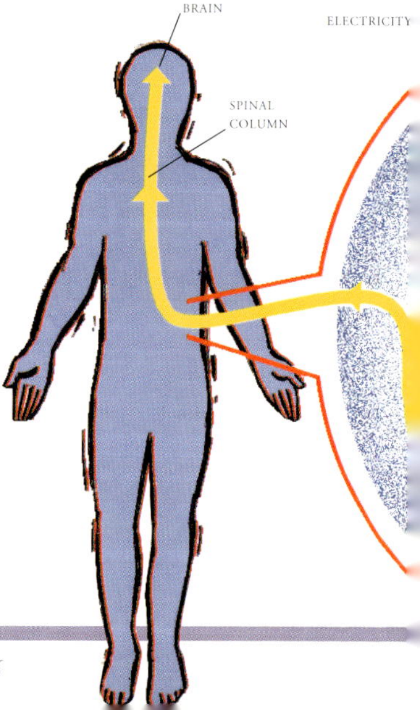

WHAT HAPPENS DURING TREATMENT?

The application of TENS is so simple that it is possible for a patient to rent or buy a device and carry out the treatment at home. A treatment lasts for about twenty minutes and can be repeated several times a day. During the session, the user can rest or continue with normal activities.

BELOW *The TENS route to pain relief by electrical impulses.*

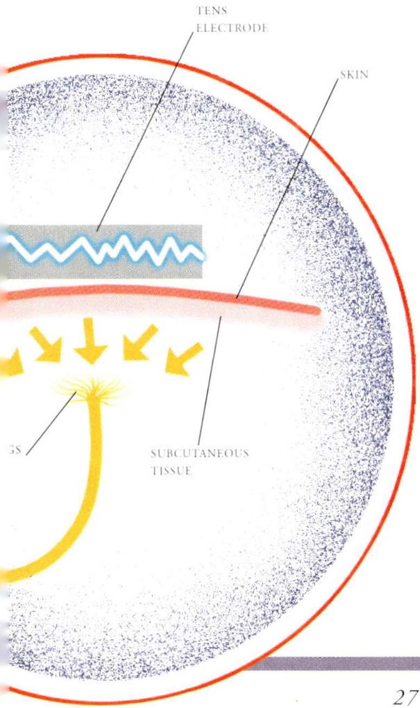

DOES IT WORK?

Numerous scientific evaluations of TENS for back pain exist. Unfortunately they do not all come to the same conclusion. But overall, TENS can play a valuable role in back pain therapy. It will often reduce the pain but rarely alleviate it totally, and it will never cure the problem altogether. Thus it is best used as an additional therapy to other effective treatment options.

GETTING OLDER

It is a fact of life that the lumbar spine becomes less flexible as we get older. Intervertebral disks wear, and distort the facet joints. Osteoporosis causes a weakening of the bones. These changes may contribute to a loss of height.

IS IT SAFE?

There is very little that can go wrong with this treatment. The TENS devices themselves are entirely safe. Very rarely, a patient might suffer an allergic skin reaction where the electrodes are attached. This irritation will quickly disappear when the TENS sessions are discontinued.

EXERCISE

Like TENS, exercise is a form of treatment used in both mainstream and complementary medicine. It is best carried out under the supervision of a well-trained therapist, such as a physiotherapist. The therapist develops an exercise program adapted to the patient's needs.

Exercise may include strengthening the muscles of the back and the trunk, as well as increasing flexibility and mobility. The intensity of the program has to be matched correctly to the progress of the patient and the symptoms.

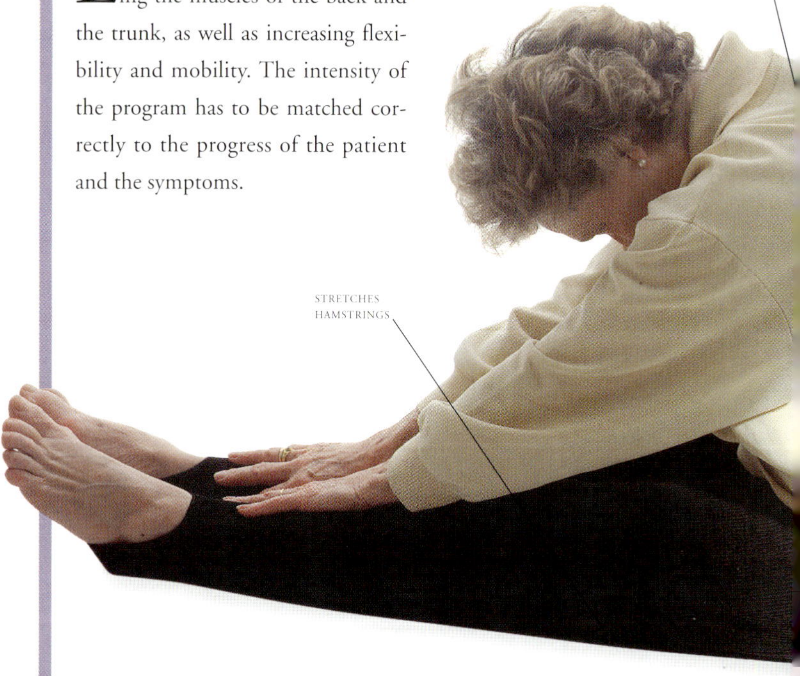

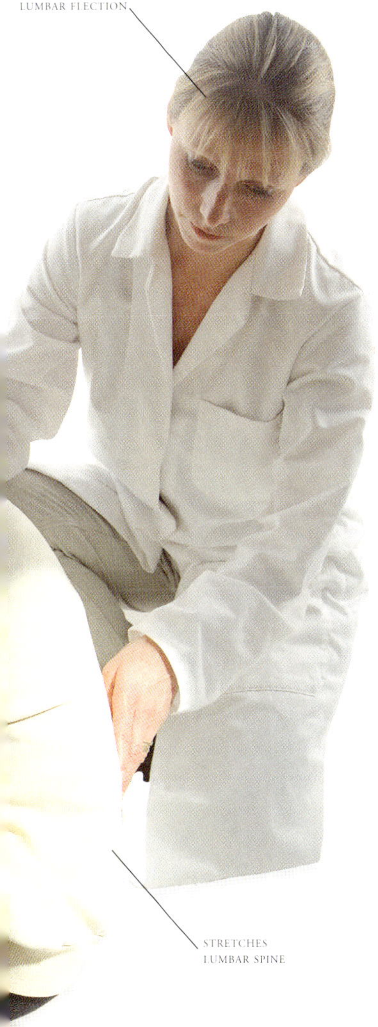

WHAT HAPPENS DURING TREATMENT?

There are various "schools" of exercise therapy. Initially the patient is carefully assessed to determine the nature of the back problem as precisely as possible. The therapist will outline suitable exercises. The patient will be asked to change into sports clothes and perform the exercises, supervised by the therapist, who will correct movements where necessary. This is important, since executing exercises wrongly may actually do some harm. It is a good idea to build up any program of exercise gradually.

To be cost-effective, small groups of patients can exercise together. A typical session will last for about half an hour. Eventually the therapist will work out an individualized home program for each patient, with exercises to repeat on a daily basis. This may be supplemented by back-friendly sports *(see page 86)*.

LEFT *Learn correct methods of exercise from a physiotherapist.*

DOES IT WORK?

There is little doubt that a well-balanced schedule of exercise is beneficial. This is borne out by the results of clinical trials as well as by everyday experience. Start with a schedule of gentle exercises. In cases of acute back pain, exercise is best started when the worst and immobilizing pain has subsided. Exercises designed to help alleviate acute symptoms also prevent chronicity. Furthermore, exercise programs have been shown to substantially reduce absenteeism from work. To ensure success, such programs should be fun, and much emphasis must be put on motivating the patients not to give up once the worst troubles are over.

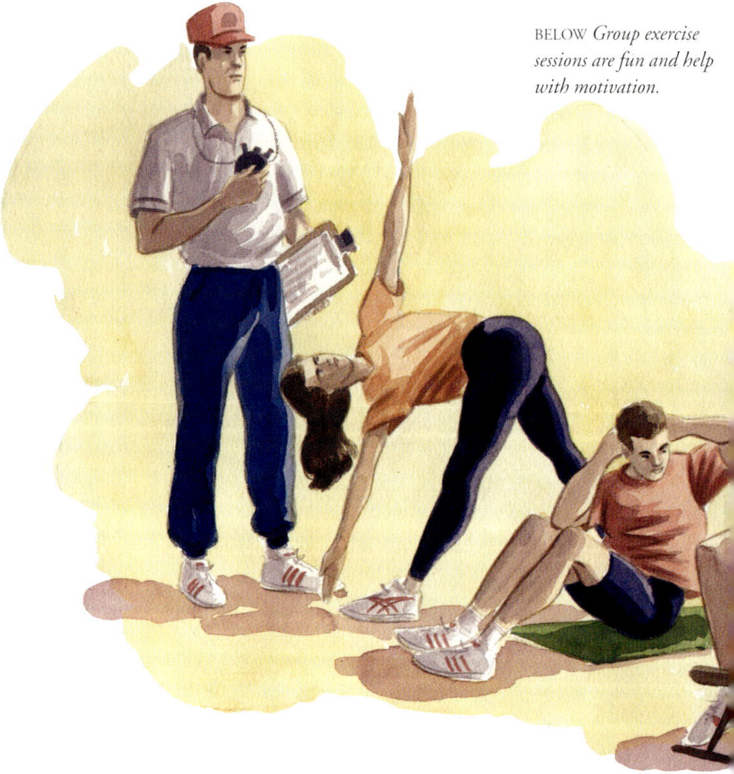

BELOW *Group exercise sessions are fun and help with motivation.*

Name Elaine Clarkson

Date June 10

Presenting symptom Pain in lumbar region for two weeks radiating into right leg.

Improvement since last session? Pain less, more localized, mobility better.

Type of exercise Flection and extension exercises, strengthening of abdominal muscles.

Frequency Daily, unsupervised.

Intensity Gently, mild only.

Duration of session Twenty minutes.

Next session In three days.

ABOVE *A patient's record from a personal treatment plan.*

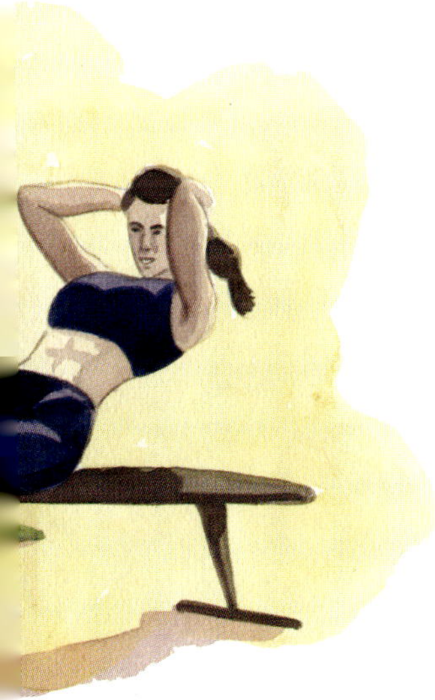

IS IT SAFE?

The wrong exercises, or the right exercises performed in the wrong way, may worsen symptoms. It is therefore mandatory that, at least initially, exercises are supervised by an experienced, well-trained therapist. Physiotherapists are the most suitable people to do this.

SPINAL MANIPULATION

CHIROPRACTIC/OSTEOPATHY

Spinal manipulation is an ancient form of treatment. In Western medical tradition, "bone setters" have long been an established part of folk medicine. Today, two main schools of spinal manipulative therapy exist in parallel: chiropractic and osteopathy.

THE HISTORY

Chiropractic was developed in the late nineteenth century by Daniel David Palmer, in the US. Apparently, Palmer cured a janitor suffering from deafness, by manipulating his cervical spine. Palmer developed a theory which suggested that all disease was caused by "malalignment" of the spine, and could therefore be cured through spinal manipulation which adjusted such "malalignment."

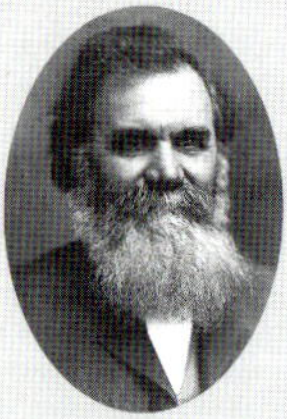

ABOVE *Daniel David Palmer developed chiropractic by manipulating the spine.*

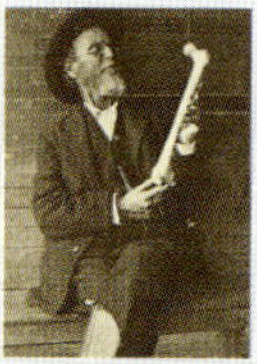

ABOVE *Andrew Taylor Still, the inventor of osteopathy.*

Osteopathy was developed around the same time in the US by Andrew Taylor Still. He too believed that spinal malfunction was at the center of all causes of disease. His original theories have a strong mystical touch and were influenced by his devout Christian beliefs.

Both schools soon acquired followers, but the theories were highly disputed by the orthodox medical profession. A battle over recognition ensued and lasted for much of the first half of the twentieth century. In recent years, chiropractic and osteopathy have become much more accepted, not least because both the schools of thought have given up the majority of their indefensible theories, and also because of emerging evidence supporting their usefulness for certain conditions. Today, chiropractic and osteopathy have gained statutory regulation in the UK. In the US, chiropractors are widely accepted by mainstream medicine, while osteopaths even have a status similar to regular physicians.

Despite the fact that historically, chiropractic and osteopathy come from different roots and constitute two separate professions, there are many similarities between both approaches .

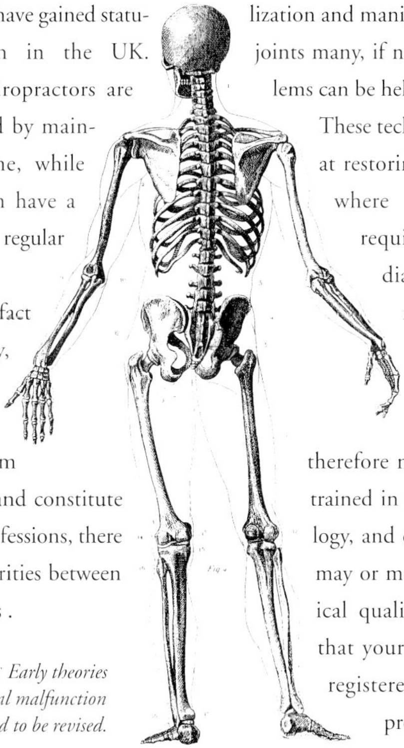

RIGHT *Early theories about spinal malfunction had to be revised.*

THE CONCEPT

Chiropractors and osteopaths had to accept that, contrary to the original theories, not all (in fact very few) diseases are caused by spinal malfunction. Today, they focus on conditions directly related to the spine. Back pain is their main area of expertise. They believe that through mobilization and manipulation of spinal joints many, if not all, back problems can be helped.

These techniques are aimed at restoring joint function where it is impaired, requiring a careful diagnostic assessment of the spinal segments.

Chiropractors and osteopaths therefore need to be highly trained in anatomy, physiology, and diagnostics. They may or may not have medical qualifications. Check that your practitioner is a registered member of a professional body.

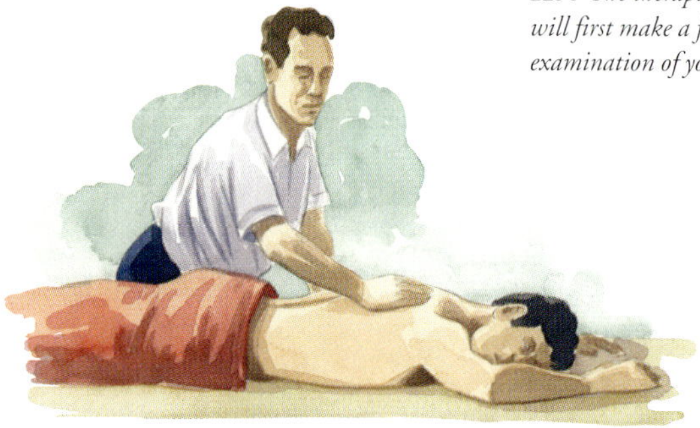

LEFT *The therapist will first make a full examination of your spine.*

WHAT HAPPENS DURING TREATMENT?

The therapist will ask about the history of your back problem, then do a thorough physical investigation. You will be asked to lie on a treatment bench and the therapist will carefully palpate the spine to test for segments of limited mobility.

The actual treatment by a chiropractor is likely to include "high-velocity thrusts" that force a joint into its full physiological range of movement. Osteopaths tend to use less forceful techniques, often concentrating on the soft tissues around the spine. Both professions will also advise you on lifestyle, bed rest, correct posture, and so on. Chiropractors are particularly likely to carry out X-ray investigations (see "Is it safe?").

A treatment session will last for twenty to thirty minutes. Normally the client does not experience pain as a result of the treatment. One treatment is rarely enough for a full recovery. Quite often, there is already some improvement after the initial session. However, pain may recur and a typical program will consist of around ten treatments carried out between one and three times per week. The therapist will then tell you to return if and when you experience back pain again. Thus several series of treatments per year are not unusual for people with chronic back problems.

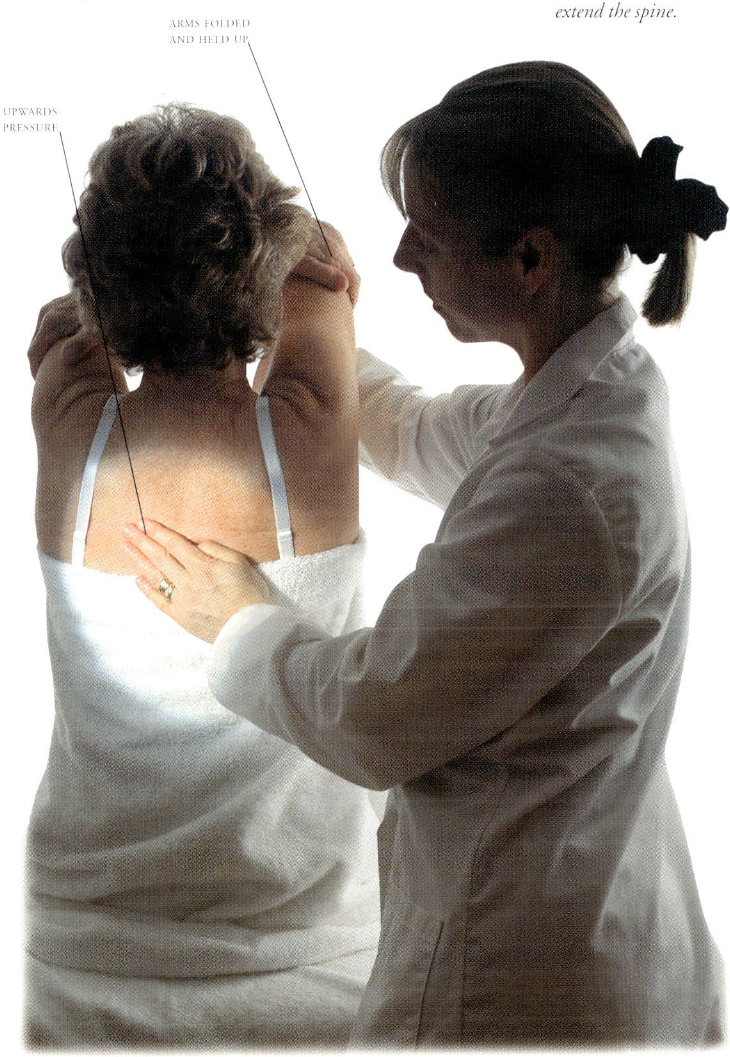

BELOW *An osteopath works to extend the spine.*

DOES IT WORK?

Many back pain patients experience significant relief from chiropractic and osteopathy. The evidence from rigorous clinical trials provides a more detailed picture. According to the data, spinal manipulation is probably effective for acute low back pain. Under these defined circumstances, it may be slightly more effective than any other treatment. If pain persists for months, the chances that manipulation will help are much less. If back pain radiates into the legs or causes paralysis or numbness, the chances are also diminished. For pain in the upper spine and neck, there is less evidence that spinal manipulation is helpful. There is little reason to suspect that one school is more successful than the other.

MANIPULATION NOTES

If possible, seek manipulation treatment early on during an episode of back pain

✧

Good for treating acute back pain

✧

Acupuncture is probably better for chronic back pain

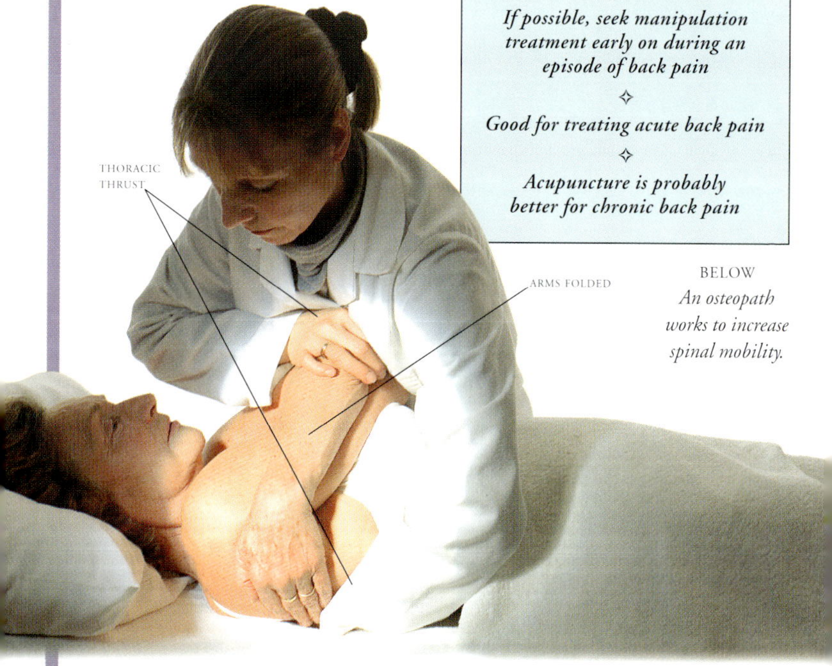

BELOW
An osteopath works to increase spinal mobility.

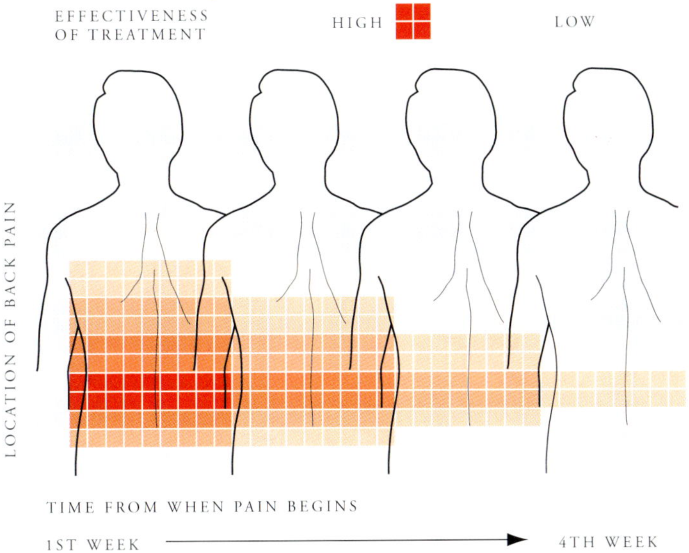

ABOVE *The graph shows low back pain is treated most successfully soon after it comes on.*

The bottom line therefore is that spinal manipulation is best tried early on during an episode of low back pain. As most such episodes last for several days only, make an appointment with a practitioner if the pain has not vanished spontaneously at the end of one week.

RESEARCH

The best evidence available today indicates that spinal manipulation is roughly as effective as acupuncture in easing back pain. While spinal manipulation is best for acute cases, acupuncture is probably better for chronic pain.

IS IT SAFE?

Contrary to what is often said, spinal manipulation is by no means free of risks. In particular, upper spinal manipulation has been associated with serious complications. With certain extreme movements, the arteries that run along the spine to the brain can be damaged. This can result in a stroke, which may even be fatal. Numerous such cases have been documented in medical literature. As with other complications of complementary therapies, we do not know how often such events occur. Considering that treatments are highly popular, one can assume that serious complications are true rarities, and spinal manipulation techniques are relatively safe.

However, there are other reasons for concern, such as the over-use of X-rays by chiropractors.' X-rays can cause cancer and therefore should be used only when truly necessary.

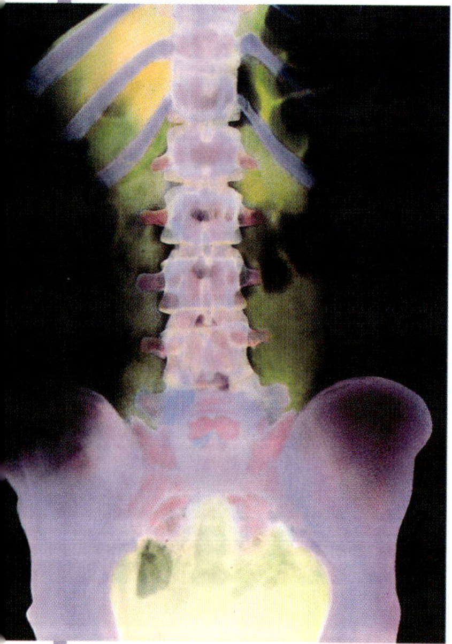

X-RAYS

Chiropractors X-ray almost every patient with back problems, often repeatedly. Many would argue that this does not provide essential information. There is no firm evidence for the presence or absence of a causal relationship between X-ray findings and back pain. X-rays are therefore unnecessarily expensive and most importantly, put patients at risk. Also, an X-ray will not necessarily show problems with muscles, ligaments, disks and nerves.

LEFT *A normal lumbar spine and pelvis. The yellow regions are soft tissue.*

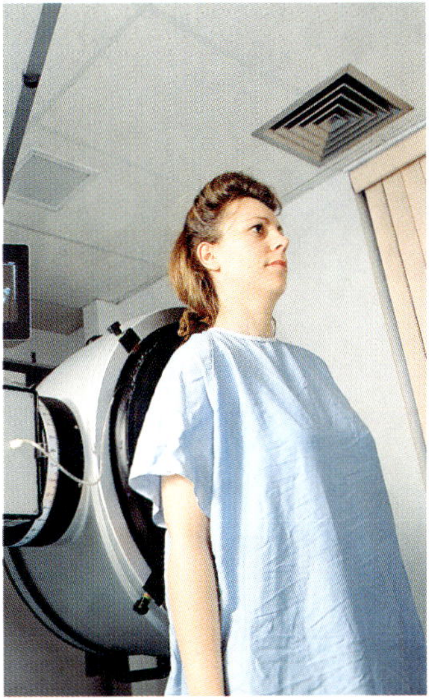

LEFT *Scanning the spine with a SPECT scanner enables the body to be viewed in slices.*

HOSPITAL INVESTIGATIONS

A specialist may request a CT or MRI scan, or a myelogram, where dye is injected into the spine to show up any nerve abnormalities.

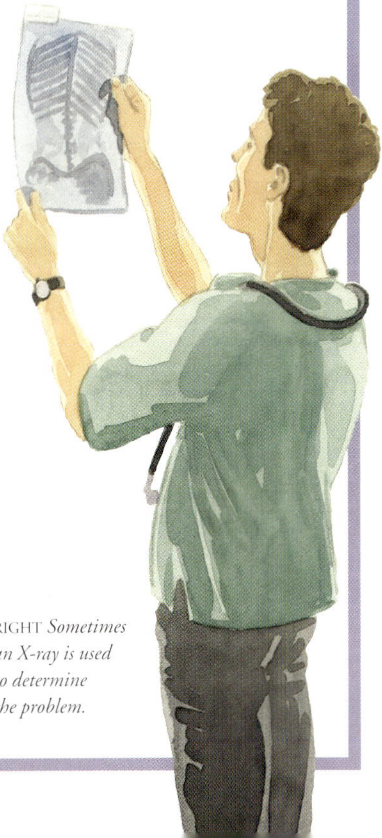

RIGHT *Sometimes an X-ray is used to determine the problem.*

DANGER SIGNALS

There are several contraindications to the "high-velocity thrust" of chiropractic. Osteoporosis is one of them. The danger is that spinal bones may fracture during chiropractic treatment, if they are brittle with osteoporosis. After the menopause, many women suffer from osteoporosis: they should therefore take a cautious approach to chiropractic. Some chiropractors think that their X-ray diagnosis can exclude osteoporosis. This is, however, a dangerous fallacy.

ACUPUNCTURE

Acupuncture has been used in China for thousands of years. It is one important element of Chinese medicine, but by no means the only one. Traditionally it would be used together with herbal treatments, exercise, massage, dietary therapies and other lifestyle approaches.

Acupuncture became widely known in the West after President Nixon's visit to China in the 1970s, when one of his staff had to have an operation and acupuncture was used as an anesthetic. Since then, its popularity has boomed and it has been subjected to rigorous scientific investigation.

THE CONCEPT

The Chinese believe that two "vital life forces" exist: Yin and Yang. If these are "out of balance" we fall ill, and treatment of any condition aims to re-balance Yin and Yang.

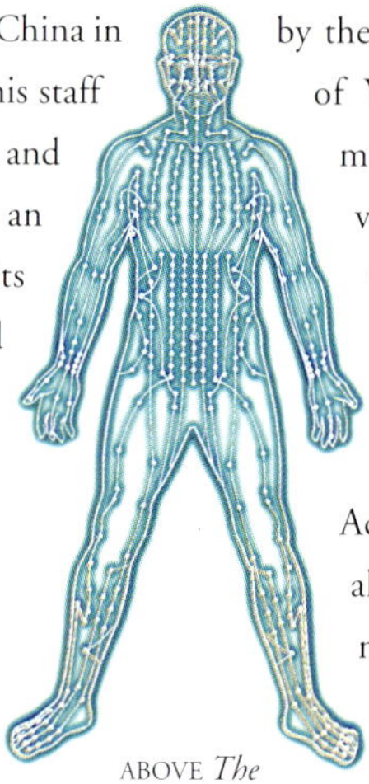

ABOVE *The meridians.*

The exact treatment schedule is not determined by the condition, but by the sufferer's unique imbalance of Yin and Yang. In Chinese medicine, treatments are individual to the patient. So a Chinese acupuncturist treating two different people suffering from back pain, may needle different points. Acupuncture points occur along energy channels, called meridians, and bear a particular relation to the life forces and to inner organs. It should be mentioned that Yin and Yang, meridians, and acupuncture points are concepts that (so far) have not been verified by modern science.

YIN AND YANG

yin is **dark**	yang is **light**
yin is **female**	yang is **male**
yin is the **earth**	yang is the **heaven**
yin is **cold**	yang is **hot**
yin is the **moon**	yang is the **sun**
yin is the **winter**	yang is the **summer**
yin is the **night**	yang is the **day**
yin is **damp**	yang is **dry**
yin is **passive**	yang is **active**

ABOVE *Yin and Yang have various attributes. The organs of the body are also principally Yin or Yang.*

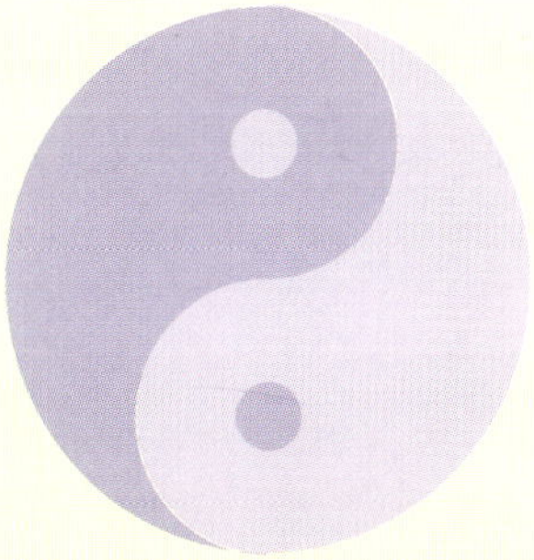

ABOVE *Yin and Yang are represented as mutually interdependent.*

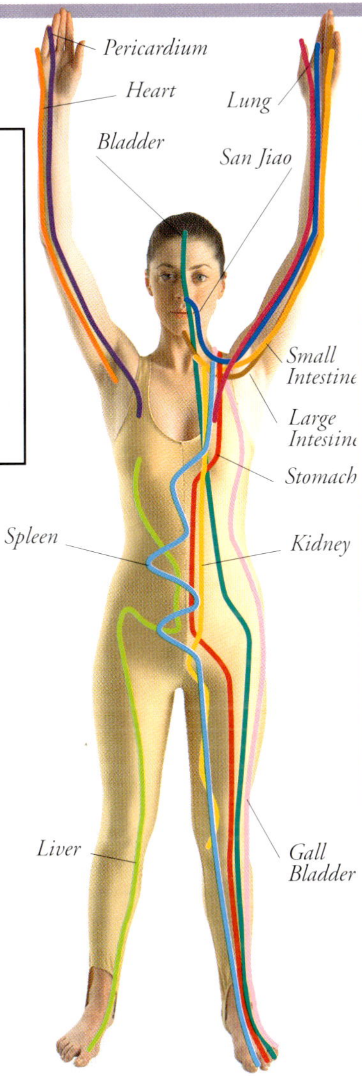

ABOVE *The meridians: invisible energy channels in the body.*

WHAT HAPPENS DURING THERAPY?

A Chinese acupuncturist (who may or may not be medically qualified) first makes a traditional Chinese diagnosis. This may involve taking a history, looking at your tongue, and feeling your pulse. Acupuncture may be one of several treatments (such as herbs, massage, or changes to the diet) suggested. To receive acupuncture, you normally lie down and several needles are placed into various acupuncture points. These points can be on the ear (auricular acupuncture) but more often those used are distributed all over your body.

The needles can be "stimulated" by hand or by connecting them to an electrical current. Sometimes heat or laser energy is used instead of the needles. The actual therapy might take around fifteen minutes.

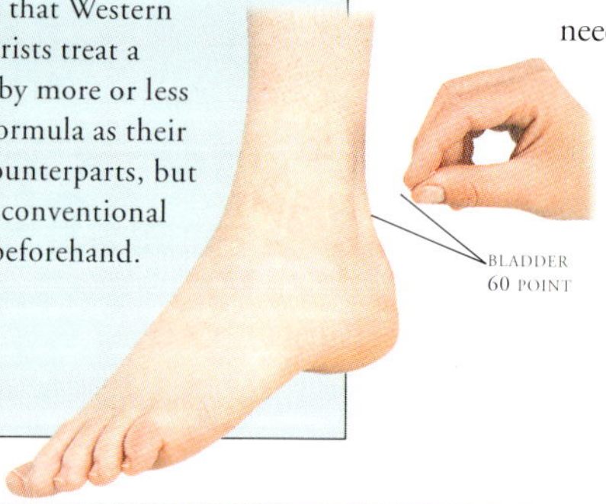

LEFT *Needling a point on the Bladder channel helps relieve lower back pain.*

WESTERN APPROACH

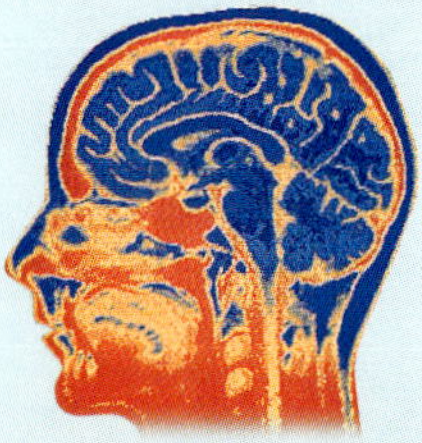

ABOVE *Acupuncture increases the level of endorphins in the brain.*

Since acupuncture was adopted by people trained in Western science, a new style has developed: Western (or medical or scientific) acupuncture. People who practice this way do not believe in Yin and Yang, or meridians. They think that the effects of acupuncture can be explained on the basis of modern neurophysiology. For instance, research has shown that after acupuncture, the concentration of endorphins (the body's own painkillers) in the brain is increased. In practical terms, this means that Western acupuncturists treat a condition by more or less the same formula as their Chinese counterparts, but insist on a conventional diagnosis beforehand.

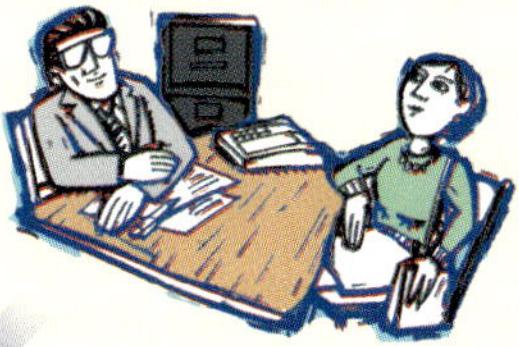

CONSULTATION
WITH PHYSICIAN

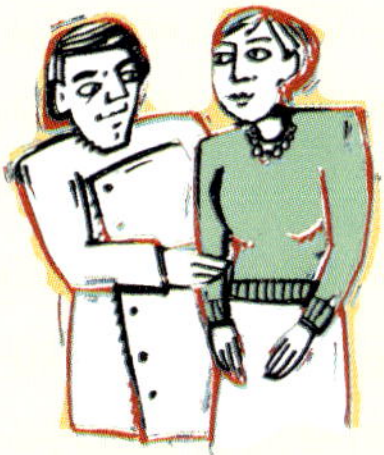

WESTERN ACUPUNCTURE

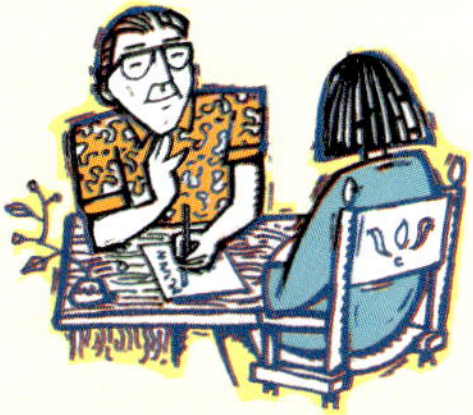

CHINESE ACUPUNCTURE

WESTERN ACUPUNCTUR

Conventional diagnosis

✧

Does not recognize concepts of Yin and Yang, or meridians

CHINESE ACUPUNCTURE

Chinese diagnosis

✧

Treatment addresses an imbalance of Yin and Yang, and meridians are needled

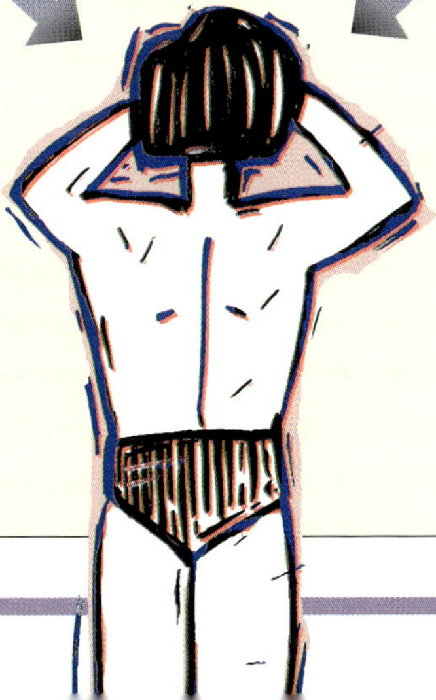

THE ACUPUNCTURE

Most patients are concerned that acupuncture will hurt. It varies: some techniques are completely painless; occasionally the needles do cause some pain, but only briefly. Most commonly there is a dull aching sensation, difficult to describe, but not unpleasant. Then the needles are removed and the session is over. Several sessions (usually six to ten) are needed for a complete course of treatment. The acupuncturist might want to see you daily, but more often treatments are carried out one to three times a week.

Typically, the Western acupuncturist is a physician and diagnoses your condition in the usual way, also examining you for tender areas. The points to be treated are chosen according to this diagnosis. The rest of the sequence of events is similar to that in Chinese acupuncture. A Western acupuncturist will often combine acupuncture with other (orthodox) treatments.

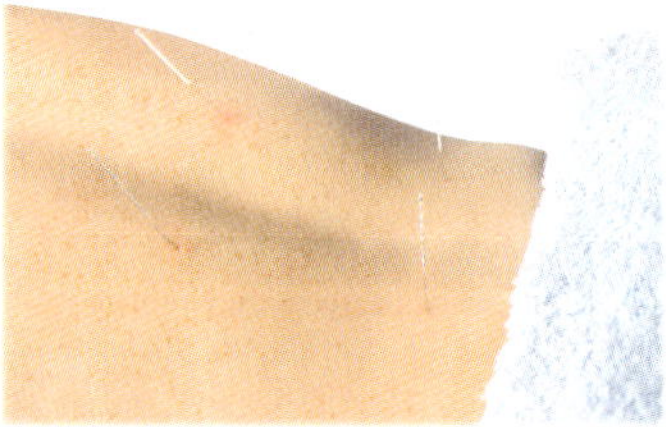

ABOVE *Needling Bladder 20 (top) and Bladder 23 (bottom). In certain places, needles are angled to prevent them going in too far, for safety. Here the lungs have been protected.*

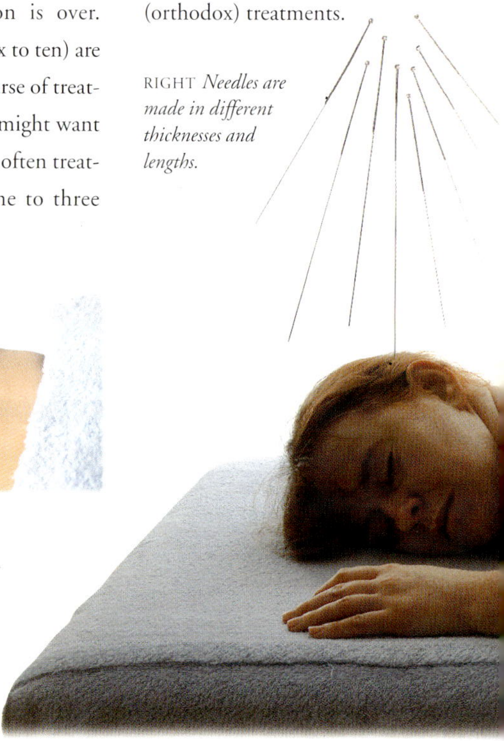

RIGHT *Needles are made in different thicknesses and lengths.*

BELOW *Working the Bladder channel helps lower back pain.*

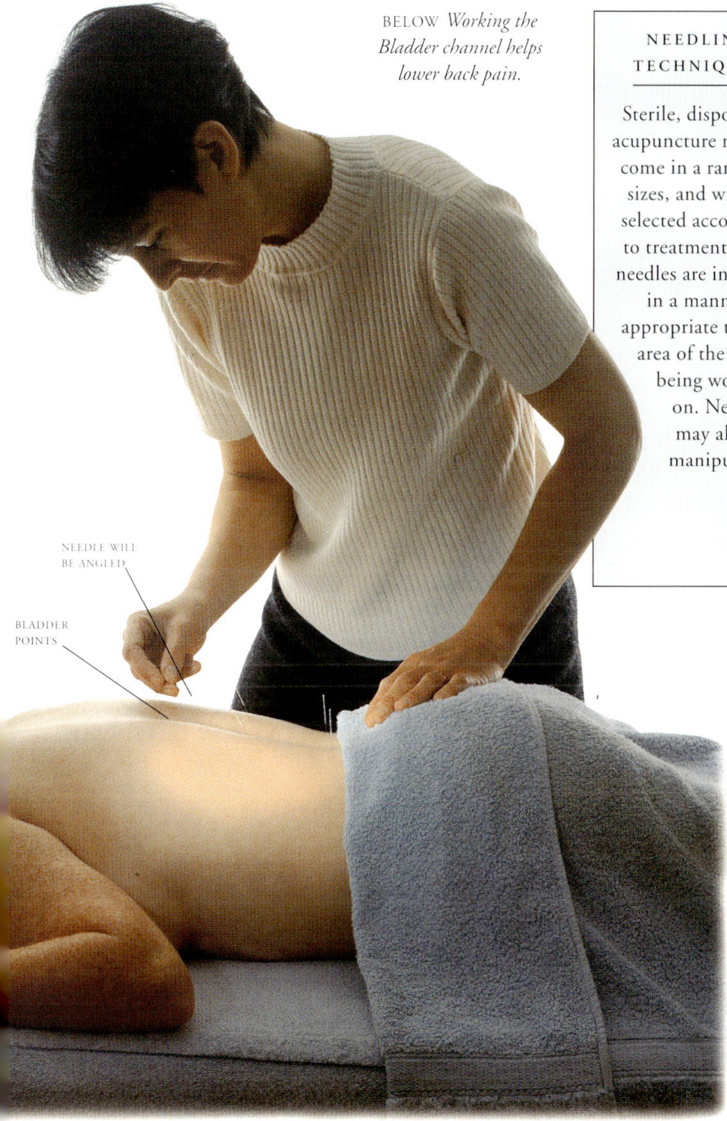

NEEDLING TECHNIQUES

Sterile, disposable acupuncture needles come in a range of sizes, and will be selected according to treatment. The needles are inserted in a manner appropriate to the area of the body being worked on. Needles may also be manipulated.

DOES IT WORK?

Many people find that their back pain is significantly improved through acupuncture. Today, most physicians accept that it can be beneficial, but the results of rigorous clinical trials are not quite as straightforward. This is partly because it is difficult to determine whether the benefit is brought about by the expectation or hope of getting better, or by the actual needles.

Despite these problems, a number of trials have attempted to find out whether the needles have a genuine effect. Most, but not all, of these suggest that acupuncture successfully relieves back pain in a significant and specific way. If the data is pooled together, the overall result is positive. Essentially this means that, based on the best evidence to date, we can state with some confidence that acupuncture is more effective than a placebo or sham acupuncture (i.e. sticking needles into random points) in reducing back pain.

CASE STUDY

Joanna Wood was a keen sportswoman during time off from her demanding job as press officer for a large company. She regularly played tennis and golf. After one particularly strenuous game of tennis, she began to suffer from a nagging pain in her upper back and shoulder. A friend recommended that she should see an acupuncturist without further delay, as this was likely to lessen the number of treatments needed, so she made an appointment for the next day.

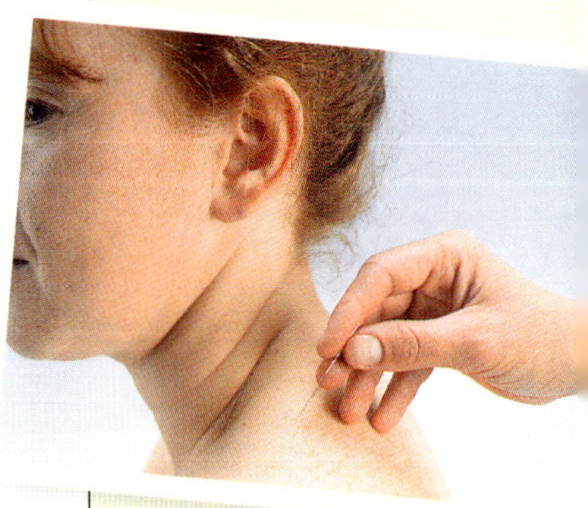

ABOVE *An upper back injury may be treated via Gall Bladder 21.*

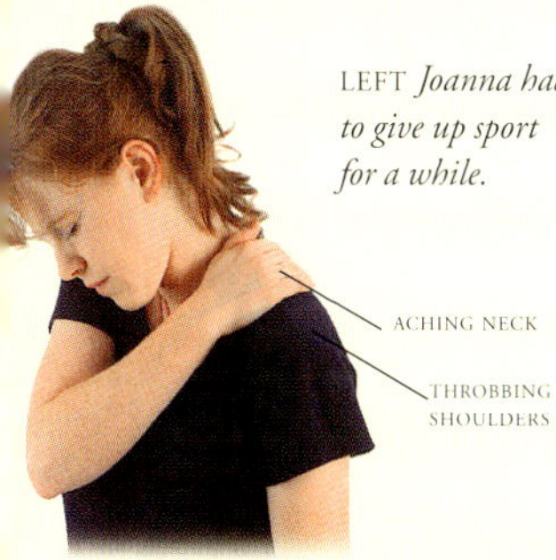

LEFT *Joanna had to give up sport for a while.*

The acupuncturist treated the Gall Bladder channel, and suggested that when the inflammation of the shoulder had gone down, moxa (burning dried herb over specific acupuncture points) could also be used to help shift blocked energy.

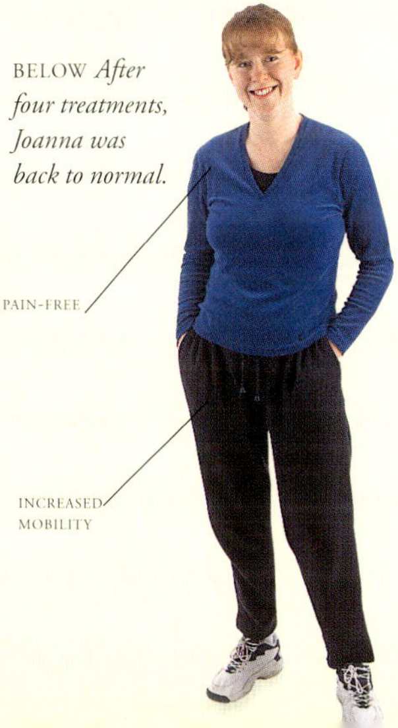

BELOW *After four treatments, Joanna was back to normal.*

IS IT SAFE?

Most people will be surprised to learn that, contrary to what many books on acupuncture will tell you, serious complications have been associated with acupuncture. The most dangerous ones are trauma to inner organs and infections. Some fifty deaths following acupuncture have been documented in medical literature.

By definition, sticking a needle into the skin is trauma: the tissue beneath the skin will be damaged. Depending on where the acupuncture needles are placed, this type of trauma can be of no consequence at all, or it can lead to dramatic complications, if for instance a needle punctures a vital organ such as the heart or the lung. Non-sterile needles can, of course, transmit infections. Make absolutely sure your acupuncturist uses disposable (one-way) needles only – most will do so anyway.

Even though these complications are on record, from what we know today, they are true rarities. Choose a reputable therapist, and the risk will be virtually negligible.

MASSAGE

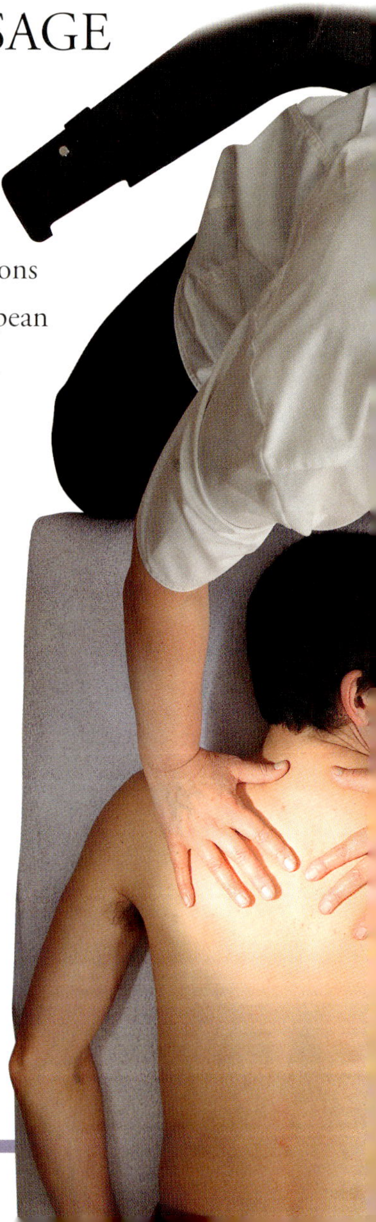

Massage is certainly one of the oldest forms of treatment known to mankind. It exists in all the major medical traditions of the world. Within the European tradition, it was forgotten and "re-invented" several times.

The most recent revival came from Sweden, and this is why the classical muscle massage techniques are sometimes called "Swedish Massage." With the discovery of potent drugs and the progress of modern biomedicine, massage was gradually pushed into the background and is now often categorized as a complementary therapy in the UK and the US. In mainland Europe, however, it is still regarded as a mainstream treatment, and most hospitals employ several massage therapists, mainly for the treatment of musculoskeletal disorders, particularly back pain.

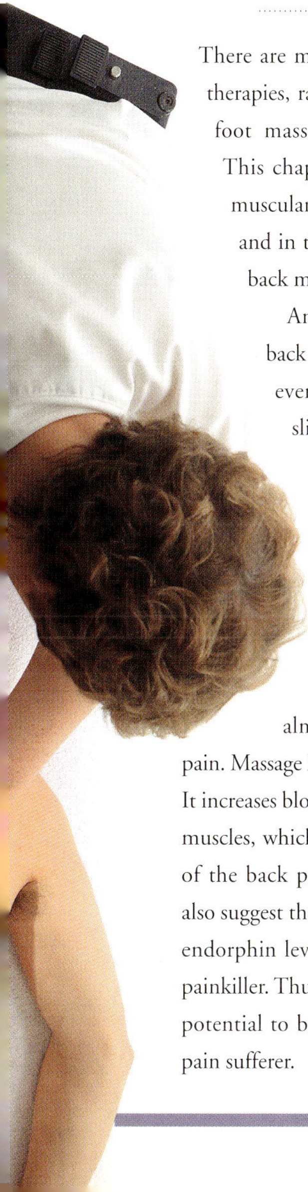

THE CONCEPT

There are many different massage therapies, ranging from Shiatsu to foot massage (see reflexology). This chapter discusses classical muscular massage techniques – and in the case of back pain, a back massage.

Anyone who has had a back massage will agree that, even though it can be slightly painful, it is also relaxing and agreeable. Back pain leads to muscular tension in the back. If done correctly, massage will relax these tensed muscles and almost instantly ease the pain. Massage has other effects as well. It increases blood flow to the skin and muscles, which can benefit the cause of the back problem. Some studies also suggest that massage can increase endorphin levels, the body's natural painkiller. Thus massage has a unique potential to bring relief to the back pain sufferer.

MASSAGE TYPES

There are numerous variations of the classical muscular massage. The list below is by no means complete:

- ✧ **Lymph drainage** is a technique of gentle stroking along the lymph vessels, aimed at increasing lymph flow and decreasing swelling.
- ✧ **Connective tissue massage** is a reflex therapy employing painful techniques which are thought to influence distant body structures via neural pathways.
- ✧ **Shiatsu** is derived from acupuncture and involves massage techniques on acupuncture points.
- ✧ **Rolfing** is forceful deep massage using hands, elbows and knuckles, aimed at releasing adhesions within the tissues around the spine.

LEFT *A back massage is a stress-buster as well as soothing painful pulled muscles.*

JOHN GREEN

First pain episode at 27, since then one episode per year. Pain after prolonged standing. No regular exercise, smoker. Has tried bed rest and painkillers.

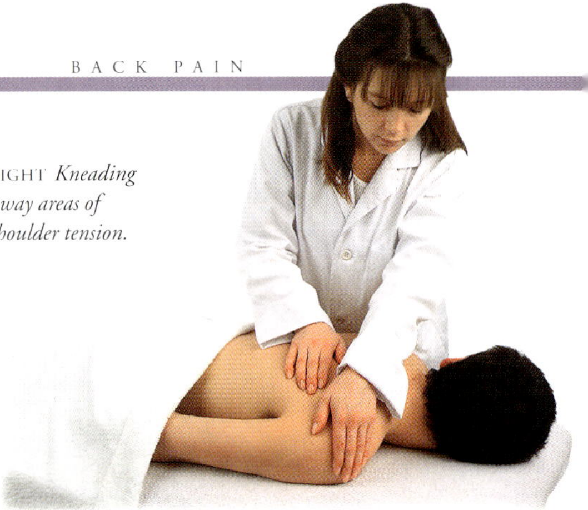

RIGHT *Kneading away areas of shoulder tension.*

WHAT HAPPENS DURING THERAPY?

A massage therapist might take a history and do a brief physical investigation. You will then be asked to undress and lie, covered with a towel, on a massage table. The massage usually starts with gentle stroking movements up and down your spine. The therapist will use a variety of techniques, some of which are targeted at deeper muscular structures. Such techniques can be mildly painful. During the course of a treatment, the therapist will find "problem areas" where your muscles are particularly knotted up. The aim is to loosen up these tender points, and this can be quite painful. The session ends with relaxing techniques. You may even drift off to sleep!

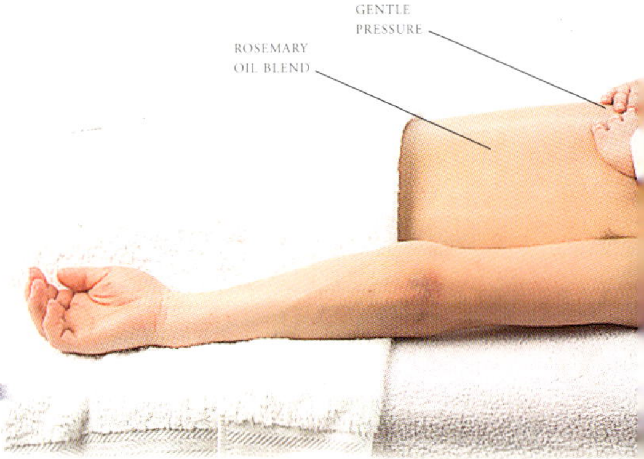

BELOW *Slow, stroking movements conclude the massage.*

One treatment usually lasts about twenty minutes. At the end of it, you may feel a marked pain relief. Yet pain will often come back when you resume your normal daily activities. Sometimes the backache is even worse than before. As the treatment is repeated, this aggravation usually wears off, and you should gradually become pain-free. A full series of treatments consists of five to ten sessions, once or twice a week.

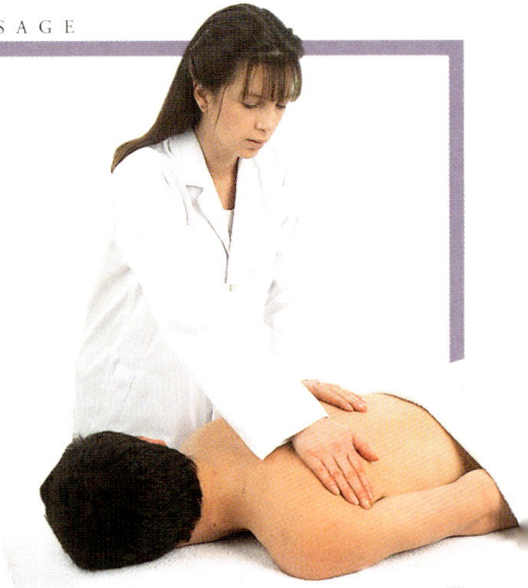

ABOVE *Pressing up each side of the torso.*

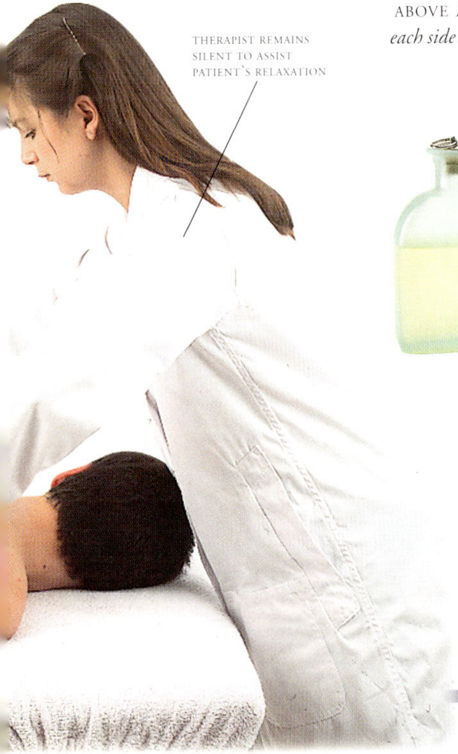

MASSAGE OILS

The oil used will be made up of a base carrier oil, such as sweet almond or grapeseed, to which a quantity of essential oil has been added. Essential oils are distilled from plants, and have various therapeutic qualities. For example, Roman chamomile is anti-inflammatory, juniper and rosemary help soothe stiff muscles.

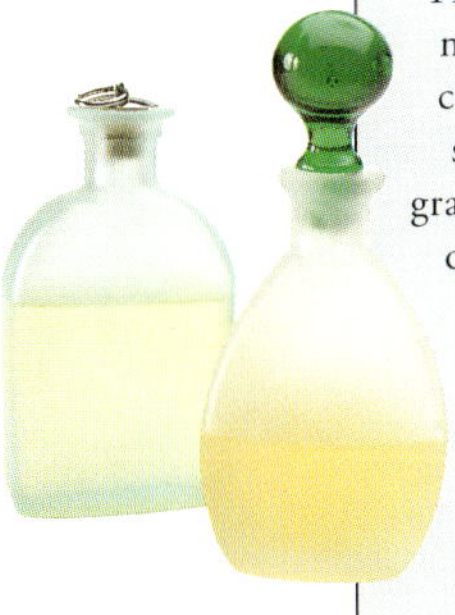

ABOVE *Black pepper oil and ginger oil blends are warming.*

DOES IT WORK?

Generally speaking, there is surprisingly little rigorous research into this particular area. Judging by my colleagues' and my own experience in prescribing massages for back pain, I have good reason to assume that it helps. Also we know about the effects massage has on the body, such as relaxation. But all this is not really compelling evidence for its efficacy in back pain.

There are only a few controlled clinical trials on the effectiveness of massage therapy. Collectively, their evidence is not entirely convincing. But this merely means that we need more evidence: it certainly does not constitute evidence against the efficacy of massage.

On balance, I believe that massage is definitely worth a try for back pain sufferers. It goes without saying that you need a therapist with whom you feel completely comfortable. Massage treatment requires rather intimate physical contact with the therapist, and this can only work if you are entirely at ease.

CASE STUDY

Mike Johnson spent the weekend clearing out his garage, moving a lot of old boxes and household items which had been stored there. By the end of Sunday night, his lower back was aching quite badly.

On Monday morning, the pain was no better after a night's rest. Mike decided to see if a massage would improve matters.

The massage therapist first asked him some general questions about his medical history.

BELOW *The wrong way to lift: bending over with straight legs.*

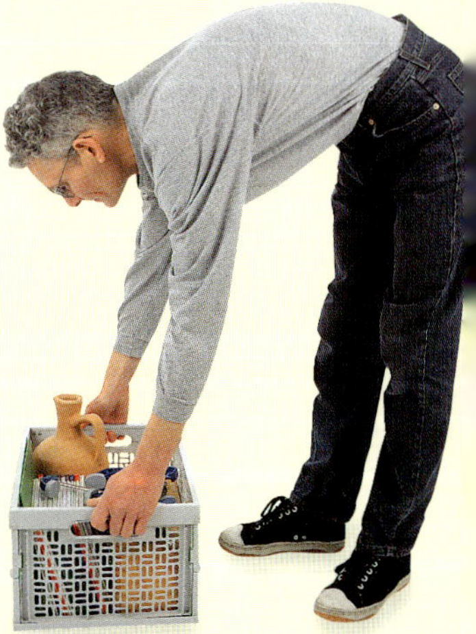

BELOW *Mike booked an early appointment before the pain got any worse.*

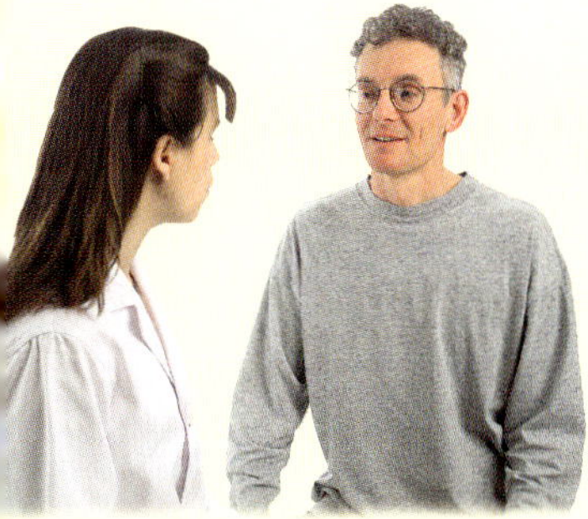

She then wanted to know exactly what had brought on the problem. Mike discovered that he had been using completely the wrong technique for lifting.

The massage therapist concentrated on massaging the whole of the back, with particular attention to the spinal muscles and the iliac crest above the buttocks.

RIGHT *Working the iliac crest, one of the painful areas.*

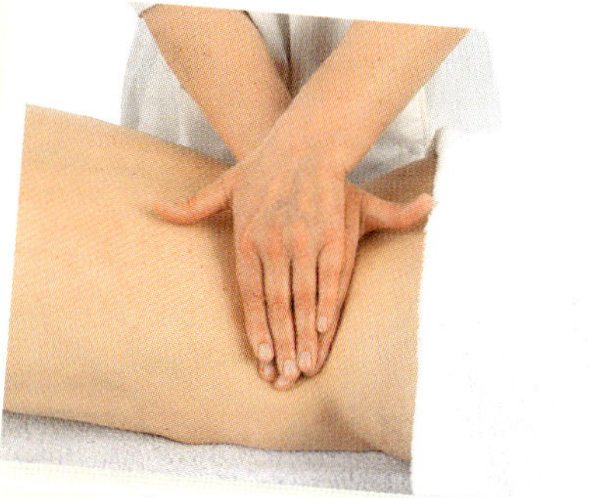

IS IT SAFE?

Yes it is. There are hardly any risks associated with massage, but avoid it in cases of dermatological diseases, open cuts or sores, heart conditions, thrombosis, tumors, varicose veins, and osteoporosis (when only gentle techniques should be used to avoid bone fractures).

Some people virtually get hooked on massage. They feel that it does them so much good that they insist on having it more and more often. While this isn't a true safety issue, it still can be harmful – not directly to the patient, but to the wallet!

THE ALEXANDER TECHNIQUE

Frederick Alexander (born 1869) was an Australian actor who suffered from voice loss which threatened his career. Through rigorous self-observation, he thought he had found the cause of his problems: incorrect body posture and movements.

Based on this concept, Alexander developed a whole system of treatment. He later moved to London where he popularized his method by running courses on it, until his death in 1955.

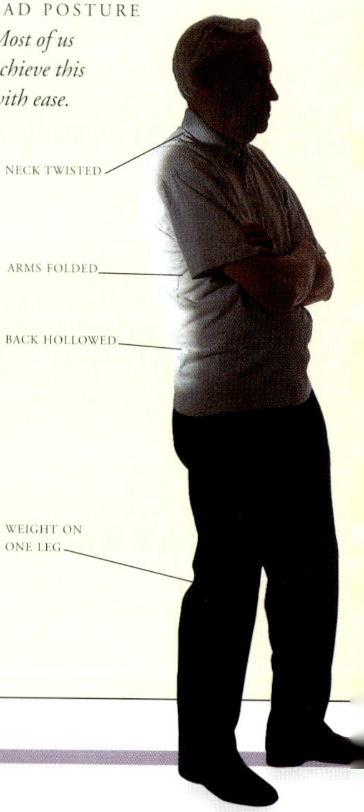

BAD POSTURE
Most of us achieve this with ease.

CORRECTING BAD HABITS

The Alexander Technique aims to teach you to "unlearn" bad habits of body posture and movement. As young children, we move with a natural grace and freedom, but this starts to disappear once we start school. The Alexander Technique is usually taught in one-to-one lessons. Each session lasts for about forty-five minutes and includes corrective exercises, the relearning of everyday activities such as sitting, standing, and walking, as well as relaxation. The lessons learned have, of course, to be followed outside classes. Alexander teachers will ensure that your body is perfectly aligned by the time you are ready to discontinue classes. It is conceivable (yet not proven) that this new strategy helps to prevent further episodes of back pain.

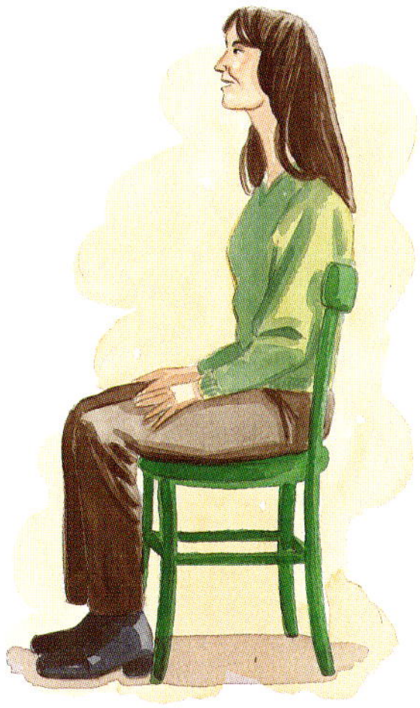

ABOVE *Sitting correctly prevents back problems starting.*

GOOD POSTURE *The Alexander Technique for standing.*

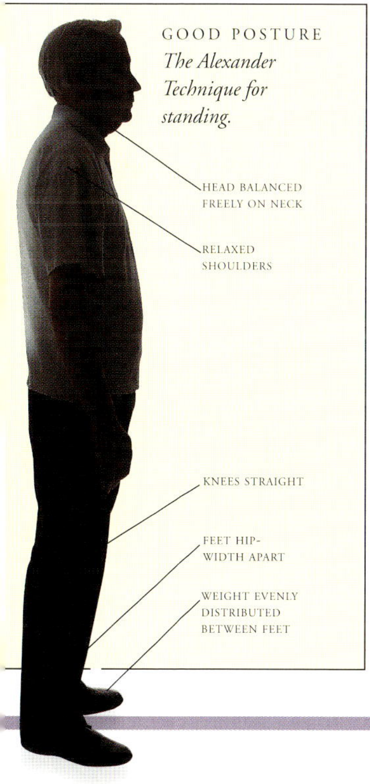

DOES IT WORK?

There has been very little research into this form of therapy. Only two clinical trials have been published, and neither of these is on back pain. The technique is, however, safe and, as some benefit is conceivable, it might be worth a try to treat and prevent back pain. The number of sessions required will depend on how quickly you are able to vanquish your bad postural habits.

HEALING

Healing (also called spiritual or faith healing) may be traced back to the New Testament (*1 Corinthians 12:9*) where it is listed amongst the gifts bestowed on the faithful. Throughout the Middle Ages, it was believed that kings and saints were given healing powers.

BELOW *Healing energy is channeled into the patient.*

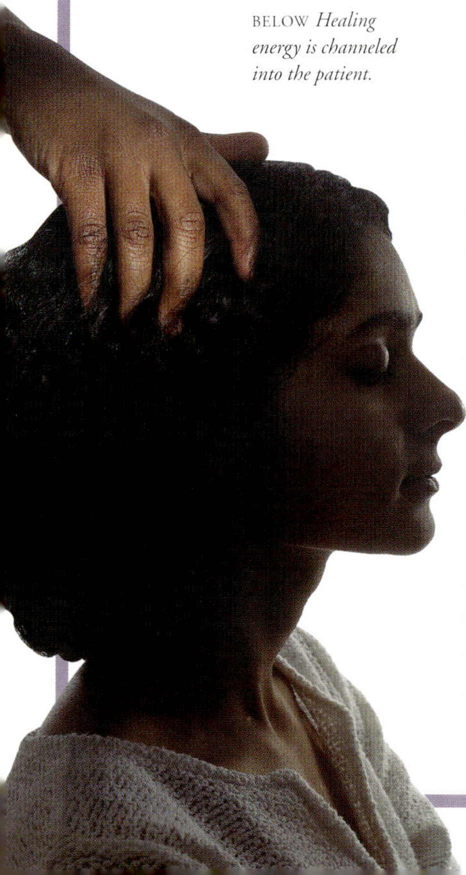

Today, healing through the "laying on of hands" (not all healers follow this method) is a widespread practice, not confined to Christian belief. In the UK, healers constitute the largest of the complementary practitioners' professions, with more than 10,000 members. Healers say that their clients do not need to believe in healing or in God.

Healers claim they can link up to an indefinable energy (sometimes called God) which enables them to cure diseases. This energy is then transmitted to the patient and cures the illness. According to healers, most health problems are amenable to healing. Pain is among the most frequent conditions treated, so it may be worth a try for back pain sufferers.

JAIRUS'S DAUGHTER

Jesus healed many illnesses. In the Bible (Luke 8:40-56), there is a well-known story about Jairus, the head of the synagogue, who begged Jesus to heal his dying daughter. When Jesus arrived at the house, the girl had died. Jesus said, "The child is not dead: she is asleep." The girl got up, fully recovered.

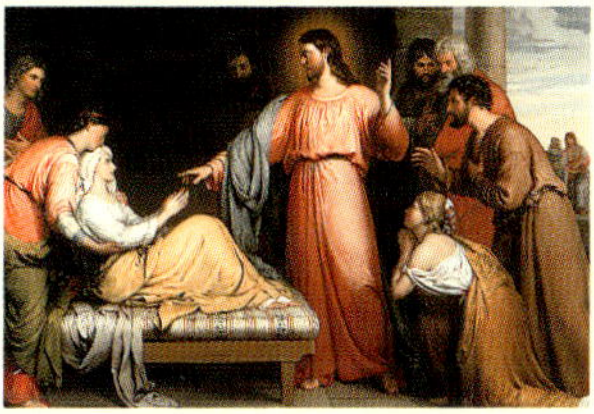

ABOVE *There are many stories of Jesus' healing miracles in the Bible.*

BELOW *Healers' powers can target pain.*

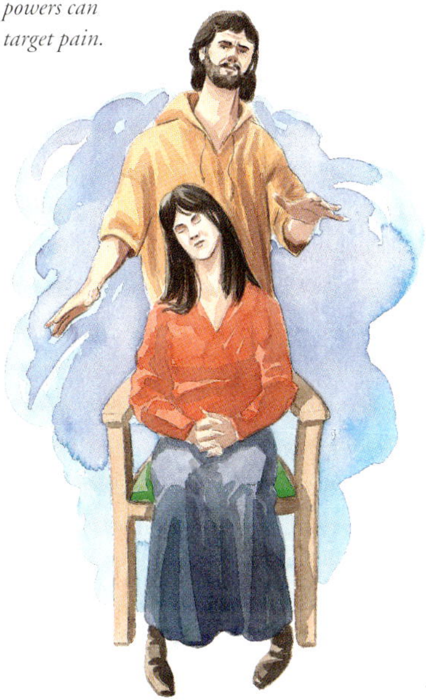

A session of healing normally requires the patient to sit or lie quietly while the healer moves his or her hands over the body, locating areas of malfunction, and then transmitting the healing energy. Many patients perceive a certain warmth in the areas under the healer's hands. A session lasts for about thirty minutes. Patients often say that they feel totally refreshed afterwards.

DOES IT WORK?

The majority of the (few) studies of healing that have been published suggest that healing does have an effect. Most are, however, burdened with methodological problems. No study of healing and back pain has been published. If done properly and with the knowledge of your physician, there is little scope for harm.

HERBALISM

The treatment of disease by plant products is called herbalism or phytotherapy. Some plant products are undoubtedly powerful drugs. Plants can kill; they can also cure or alleviate health problems. Historically, almost all our drugs have relied on plants, and herbalism is an element found in all cultures.

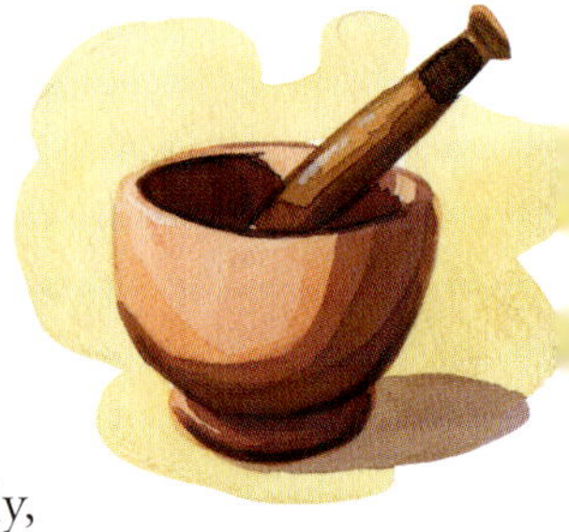

ABOVE *Herbal medicine has been used for thousands of years.*

Today, in Western society, herbalism has been driven towards the fringes of medicine, not least because of the advent of powerful modern synthetic drugs.

There are two kinds of approach: traditional herbalism and rational phytotherapy. A traditional herbalist assesses each patient in a holistic fashion, with little or no emphasis on conventional diagnoses. Herbs are then prescribed according to the individual who is being treated, rather than according to the disease or symptom. Rational phytotherapy, in contrast, uses plant extracts much like physicians use synthetic drugs: a given condition is likely to respond to a given set of plant extracts.

PLANT POWER

Several plant extracts are known to alleviate pain. In fact, the bark of the willow tree was the original material for aspirin. It contains salicylates and was traditionally used for treating pain. It was, however, burdened with nasty gastrointestinal side-effects. Thus aspirin was developed, which is more potent and has fewer side-effects than the original plant material. Another fairly well-researched example is a plant called Devil's claw (*Hapargophytum procumbens*). Clinical trials have shown it to be effective in reducing pain. Several other herbs contain various biochemicals which have analgesic or anti-inflammatory properties – see some examples in the box below.

What are the advantages of phytotherapy over conventional drug treatment? Aspirin seems to tell us the opposite, but some plants definitely have fewer side-effects than synthetic drugs. They may also be less expensive. And some people simply prefer to be treated by natural products, even though the advantage may be slight or non-existent.

PAIN-RELIEVING PLANTS

URTICA DIOICA

Nettles are a tonic for the whole body.

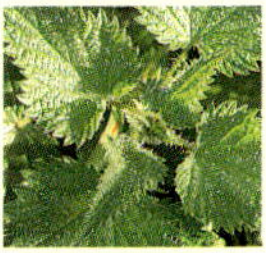

BOSWELLIA CARTERI

Frankincense resin comes from a tree.

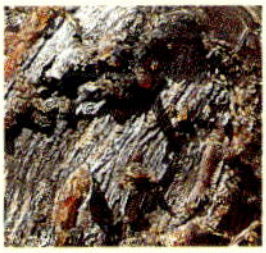

SALIX ALBA/NIGRA

Willow bark helps reduce inflammation.

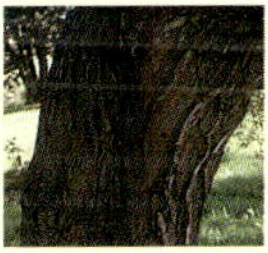

POPULUS TREMULA

Poplar bark helps pain and swelling.

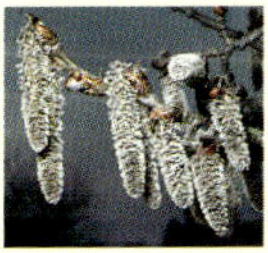

SOLIDAGO VIRGAUREA

Pick golden rod when it is in flower.

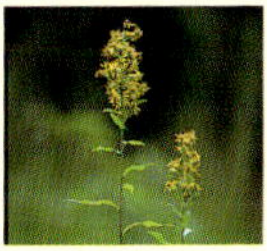

FRAXINUS EXCELSIOR

The common ash is a quick-growing tree.

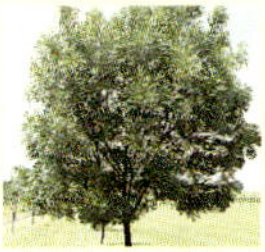

ALCHEMILLA MOLLIS

Lady's mantle flowers and leaves are used.

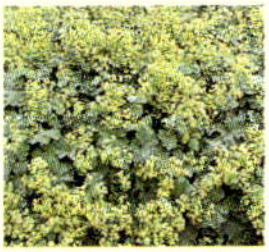

EQUISETUM ARVENSE

Horsetail's silica content helps to heal wounds.

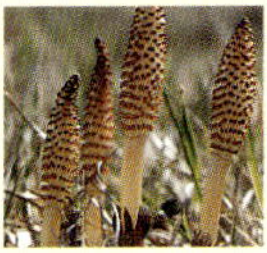

HOMEOPATHY

Homeopathy was developed by a German physician, Samuel Hahnemann (1755–1843). Hahnemann was disillusioned with the standard medical practices of the time, and began to experiment with a new system he named homeopathy, after the Greek words meaning "like" and "suffering."

Homeopathy is essentially based on two principles. The "like cures like" principle claims the following: if a given remedy causes certain symptoms (say a headache) when administered to a healthy person, this remedy can be used for a patient who suffers from headache. The second principle has it that, through the special steps of dilution applied to a substance to make a remedy, it does not become weaker but more potent. This applies even if the dilution is so great that not a single molecule of the original substance is left in the actual remedy.

Homeopathy was very popular 150 years ago. It then went out of fashion, not least because of opposition from mainstream medicine. Scientists state that where there is no molecule there can be no effect, and homeopathy's effectiveness is unproven. In spite of these arguments, it is in vogue again. Back sufferers are likely, therefore, to consider it as a treatment.

HOMEOPATHIC SUBSTANCES

BELOW *Bellis helps deep wounds such as pelvic surgery.*

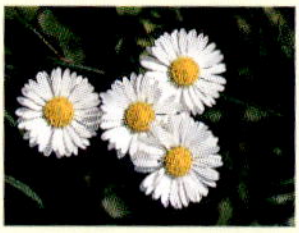

BELOW *Cimicifuga treats back pain and arthritis.*

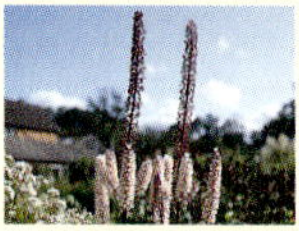

BELOW *Symphytum helps to heal broken bones.*

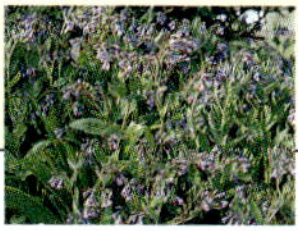

CONSULTING A HOMEOPATH

The homeopath will take your history in minute detail. At the end of this often long encounter, a remedy will be chosen that best fits your overall picture. Two different patients with back pain might receive two entirely different remedies. Critics claim that this highly empathic therapeutic encounter is the true reason for the apparent success of homeopathy. There have been more than a hundred clinical trials of homeopathy, but no research has been published in relation to back pain.

The homeopath will make notes on your:

- Personality
- Temperament
- Behavior patterns
- Moods
- Emotions
- Worries
- Fears
- Health problems

Little harm can be done by homeopathy, provided that you remain under the ultimate control of your physician. If you are inclined, give it a try. The first session might take an hour for the homeopathist to get an overall picture; following sessions are shorter.

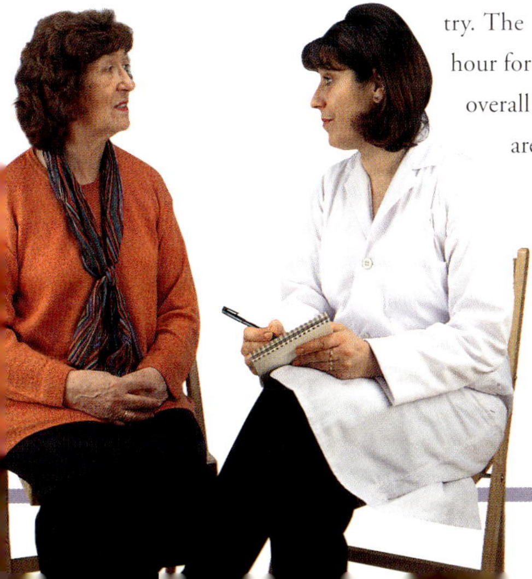

LEFT *A homeopath will build up a detailed picture.*

REFLEXOLOGY

Reflexologists believe that body parts and inner organs are represented on the sole of the foot in the form of reflex zones (the system is sometimes also called reflex zone therapy). Maps of the feet have been drawn up to show the zones and their associated body parts.

The feet are massaged in order to find areas of resistance in the subcutaneous tissues of the sole of the foot. These areas indicate the localization of malfunction within the body – simply by reference to the map of reflex zones.

Following this diagnostic step, reflexologists treat the abnormalities found by applying pressure to the sole of the foot. They believe that, once the resistance in the tissue is dissolved by massage, the malfunction of the body will also disappear.

A reflexology session therefore requires you to bare your feet and undertake some intense massage action on the soles of both feet.

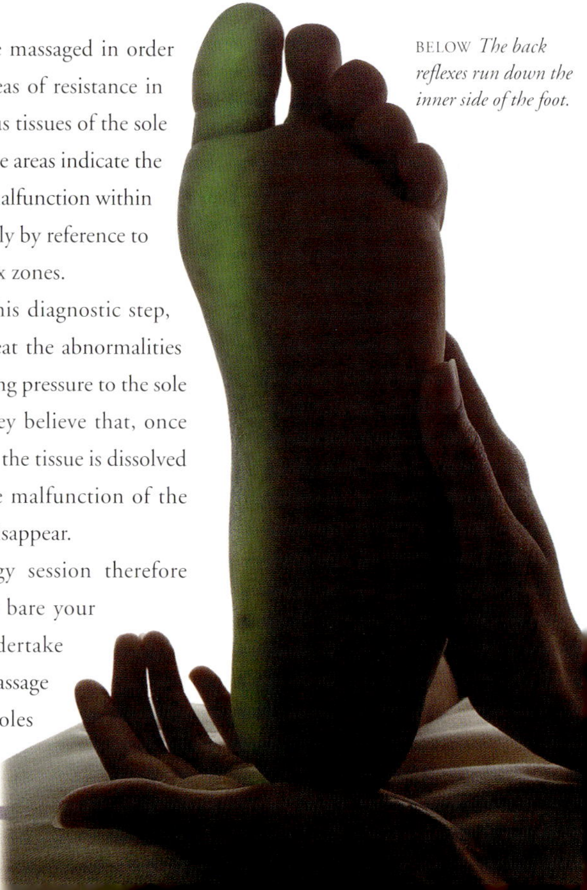

BELOW *The back reflexes run down the inner side of the foot.*

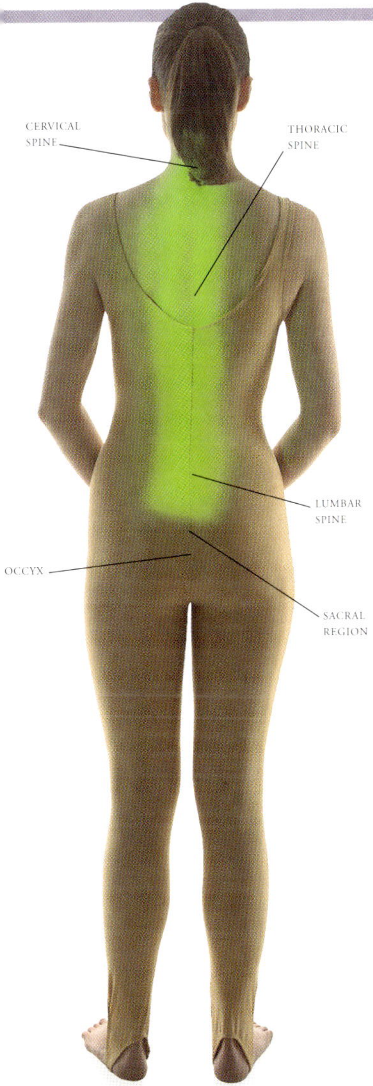

ABOVE *The related areas on the spine.*

This can be somewhat painful, but most people experience the treatment as intensely relaxing and pleasurable. A session normally lasts for about twenty minutes.

DOES IT WORK?

There is little research into this area. Our own investigations show that the diagnostic procedure of reflexologists is not reliable. Firstly, the diagnoses achieved do not correspond to validated diagnoses by physicians. Secondly, diagnoses differ almost at random among a group of (well-trained) reflexologists. There have been several clinical trials of reflexology, with both positive and negative results. To date, no trial on back pain has been published.

So it is not easy to give advice for back pain sufferers. There is certainly little scope for harm, provided you remain under the control of your physician. There is also little doubt that reflexology can be a most agreeable and relaxing experience. Usually five to ten sessions are advocated for treating an episode of back pain.

ROLFING

The American biochemist Dr Ida Rolf (1896–1976) was the "inventor" of structural integration or Rolfing. In developing this technique, she drew from other methods such as yoga, osteopathy, and the Alexander Technique.

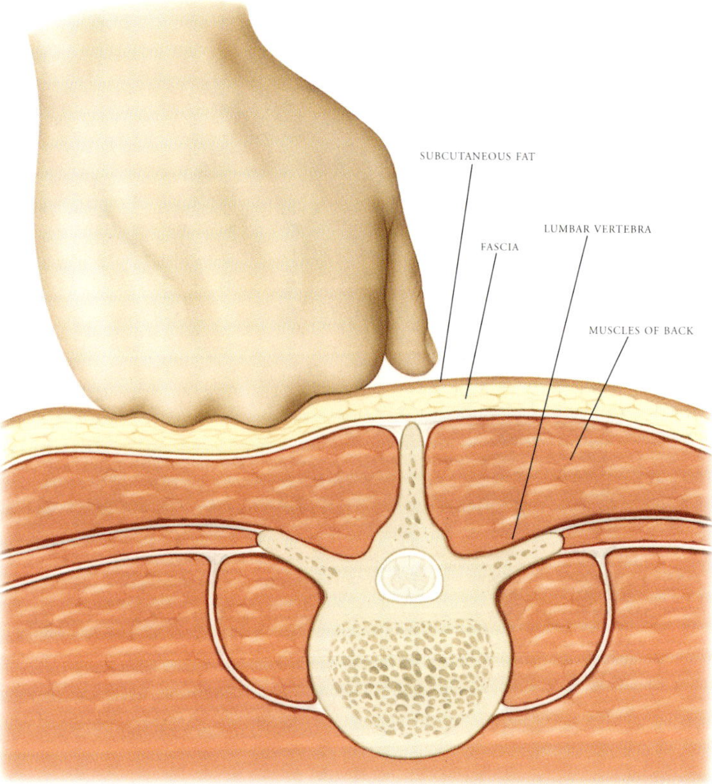

In Rolfing, the therapist applies deep pressure to the fascia, the thin layers of tissue that cover our muscles. Rolfers believe that adhesions of the fascia are responsible for faulty body alignment which, in turn, is the cause for many ailments. The therapist will see that your back gets properly aligned – by a process of correcting your posture and the interaction of your body parts.

During therapy, Rolfers use their fingers, knuckles, elbows and even knees to apply corrective pressures. Rolfing will also include an individualized program of corrective exercises. During a treatment session you will need to partly undress and lie on a massage bed for most of the time. The pressure applied by Rolfers can be intense, and the experience may be extremely painful.

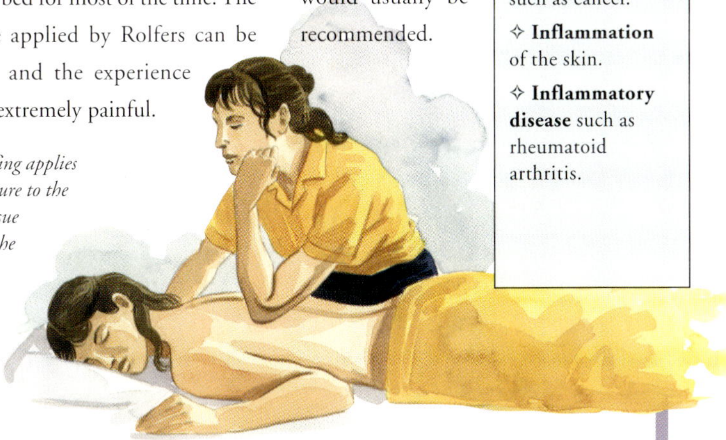

LEFT *Rolfing applies deep pressure to the fascia (tissue covering the muscles).*

DOES IT WORK?

Very little research has been done on Rolfing. No research at all has been published in relation to back pain. So it is possible that Rolfing may alleviate your back pain, but it is certainly not proven. Other than an increase in pain, there are few conceivable risks. A session lasts about thirty minutes, and five to ten sessions would usually be recommended.

CHECKLIST

Rolfing is suitable for treating:

✧ **Musculoskeletal pain** caused by mechanical stress.

✧ **Poor posture** causing poor body alignment.

Do not use rolfing when there is:

✧ **Osteoporosis**

✧ **Fracture** of a bone.

✧ **Serious disease** such as cancer.

✧ **Inflammation** of the skin.

✧ **Inflammatory disease** such as rheumatoid arthritis.

TAI CHI

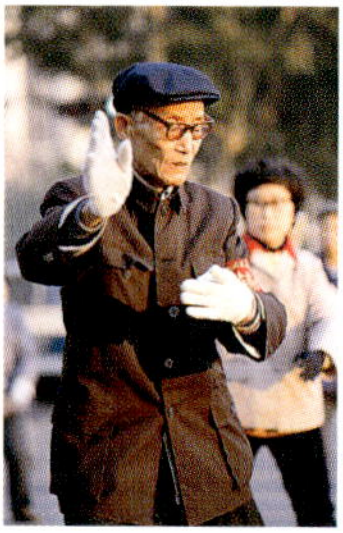

ABOVE *Elderly man in Shanghai practicing Tai Chi.*

Tai Chi is an ancient Chinese form of gentle exercise, still practiced on a daily basis by millions of (mostly elderly) people in China. It is thought to improve well-being through a program of controlled slow movements, meditation, concentration, and breathing exercises.

The philosophy of Tai Chi is to build up strength, create rhythm and balance the body's inert energy. Like acupuncture, it is firmly rooted in Taoism. Since Tai Chi has become popular in the West, it has also been investigated scientifically. Several clinical trials suggest that it does indeed convey health benefits, particularly in the elderly. One recent study of back pain sufferers also implies benefit: patients regularly following a Tai Chi program felt less pain and more mobility. They also felt more relaxed and could cope better with the residual pain.

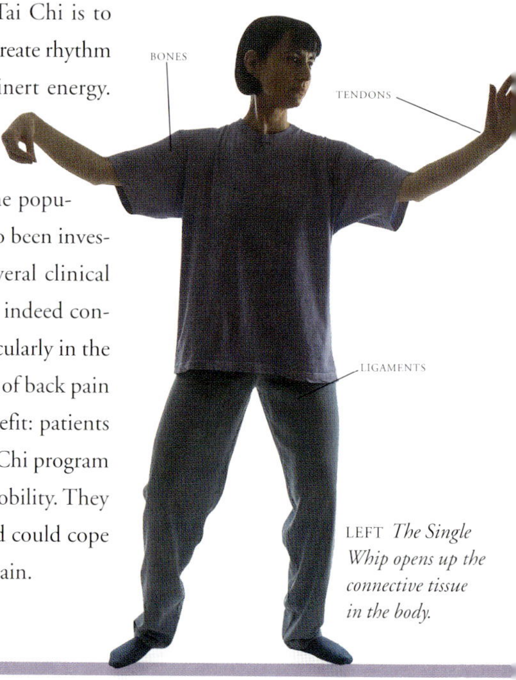

LEFT *The Single Whip opens up the connective tissue in the body.*

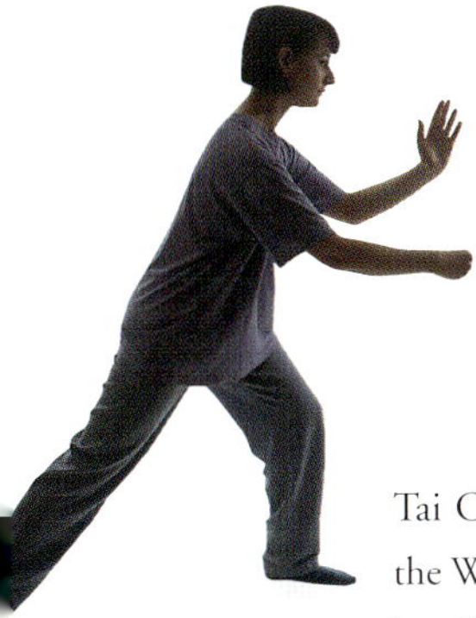

ABOVE *Punch Down will stretch the ligaments of the legs.*

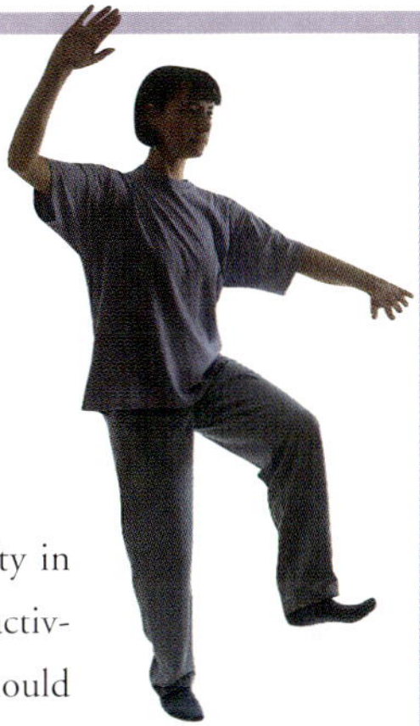

ABOVE *White Crane Spreads Wings requires good balance.*

JOIN A CLASS

Tai Chi is fast gaining popularity in the West as a health-promoting activity. If you want to try it, you should join classes and learn the technique from an experienced teacher. This can't be done quickly and should therefore be seen as a long-term investment of time. Tai Chi needs to be done every day for about half an hour. There are no conceivable serious risks in taking up Tai Chi so, provided you are interested, give it a try.

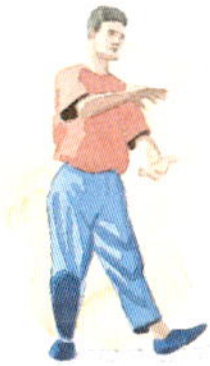

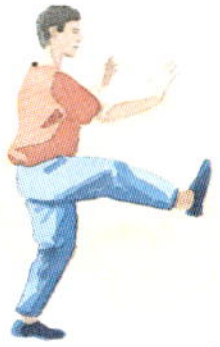

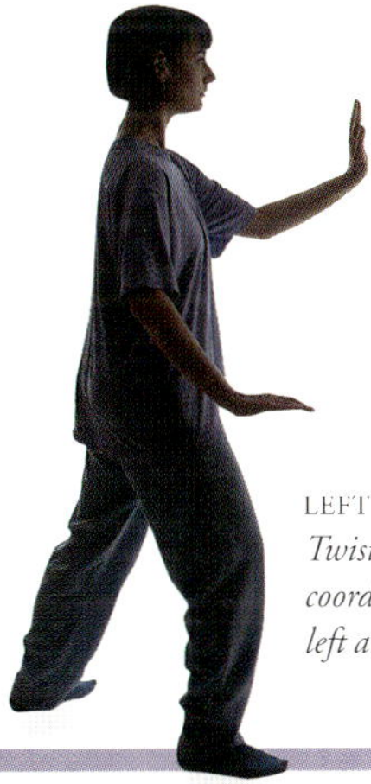

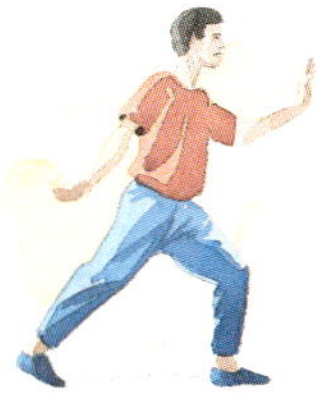

LEFT *Brush Knee And Twist Step develops coordination between left and right.*

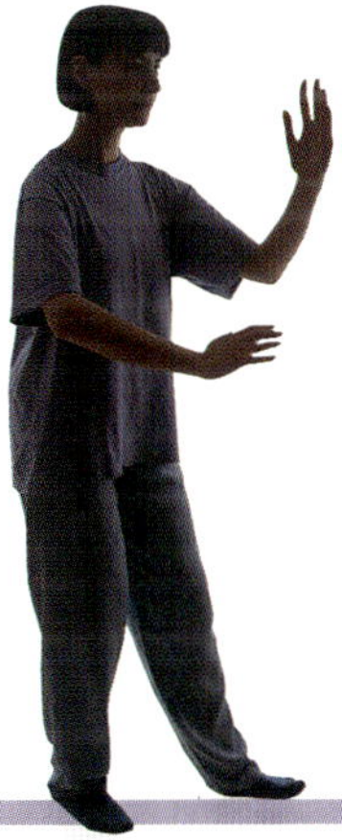

RIGHT *Play The Lute is a very graceful part of a routine.*

YOGA

Yoga is an umbrella term for several techniques involving a highly disciplined activity based on Hindu philosophy. It can comprise a set of exercises (Hatha yoga), and relaxation and breathing techniques (Prana yoga). It promotes fitness, flexibility of movement, relaxation, and general well-being.

HEALTH CHECK

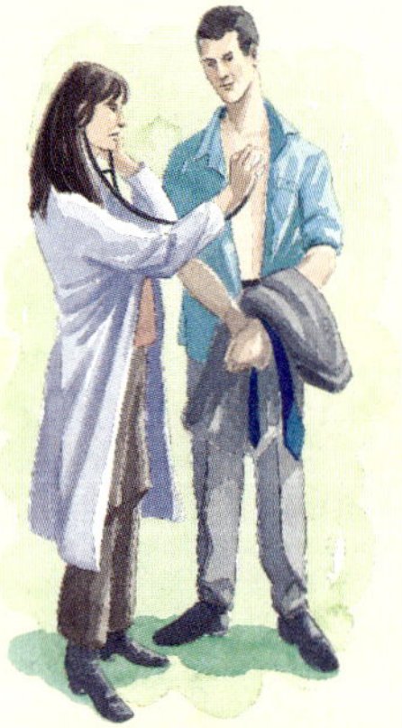

Check with your physician to make sure there are no physical problems which caution against yoga. Certain positions may be inadvisable, depending on your back problem.

Yoga has been popular in the West for some time. It can be learned from experienced teachers, either by attending a group class, or on an individual basis. This is not a quick process, so be patient and expect to invest a considerable amount of time. One session lasts up to an hour, and regular practice is required in addition.

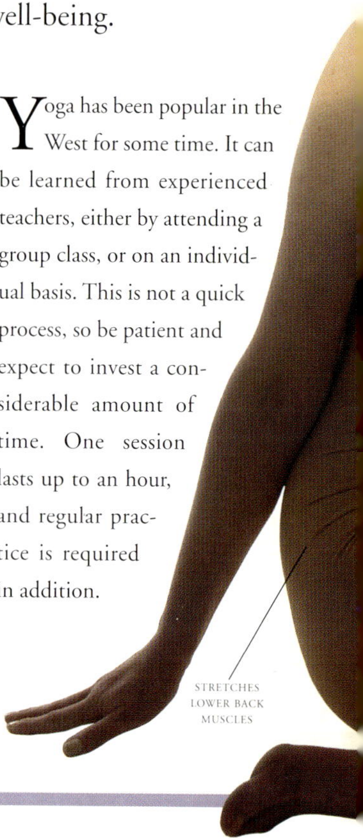

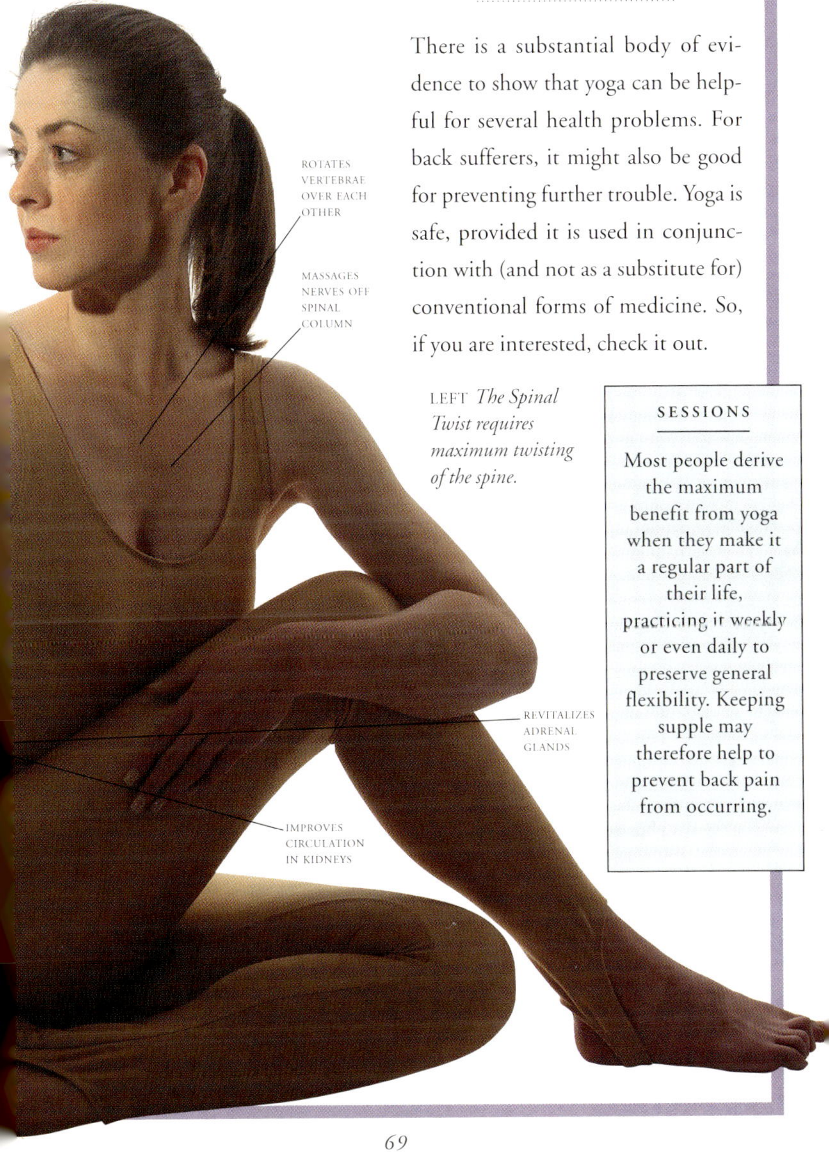

DOES IT WORK?

There is a substantial body of evidence to show that yoga can be helpful for several health problems. For back sufferers, it might also be good for preventing further trouble. Yoga is safe, provided it is used in conjunction with (and not as a substitute for) conventional forms of medicine. So, if you are interested, check it out.

LEFT *The Spinal Twist requires maximum twisting of the spine.*

SESSIONS

Most people derive the maximum benefit from yoga when they make it a regular part of their life, practicing it weekly or even daily to preserve general flexibility. Keeping supple may therefore help to prevent back pain from occurring.

CHOOSING A COMPLEMENTARY THERAPIST

When you go and see your general physician, you can be sure that he or she has studied medicine and obtained adequate experience. But complementary medicine is largely unregulated.

Unquestionably there are many highly qualified complementary practitioners, but there are also less qualified ones and charlatans.

The best way to find a good practitioner is to ask your physician to recommend one. Or ask someone you trust, who you know is critical. Make sure your practitioner is not a "greenhorn" who is just starting in the profession. Check that he or she has several years' training and belongs to a reputable professional organization.

PRACTITIONER CHECKLIST

At your first visit, take the time to ask the following questions. Don't be shy – it is for your own good.

What qualifications do you have?

How long have you practiced?

Which professional body do you belong to?

Have you got insurance cover?

Do you think that you can ease my pain?

Of what exactly does the therapy consist?

What side-effects may occur?

How many treatment sessions will be required?

How much will it cost?

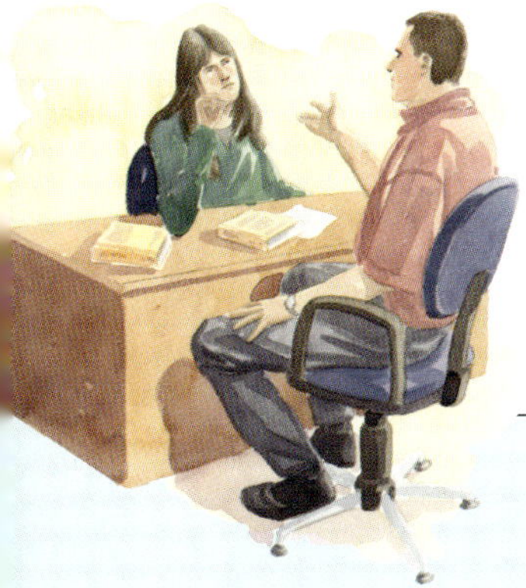

If the practitioner refuses to answer any of these questions, or if the answers do not completely satisfy you, find another therapist. Furthermore, avoid therapists who:

Interfere with your physician's prescriptions.

Promise a quick and total cure. (If it sounds too good to be true, it usually is!)

Claim that their method of treatment is the only one that will help you.

Speak badly about other healthcare professionals.

Claim that their method is free of risks.

COMBINING SEVERAL TREATMENTS

Many complementary therapies can be combined in a meaningful way. You may, for instance, use massage and exercise treatments in parallel. The massage will even make you more ready for the demands of exercise. Alternatively, you could combine spinal manipulation with acupuncture or TENS. There are virtually no rules and restrictions other than the amount in your budget.

It makes a lot of sense to combine the best of the two worlds of complementary and mainstream medicine. Always see your physician when you have back pain. Discuss the options and follow the prescription you are given. Tell your physician which complementary therapies you are considering in addition to the treatment he or she advises, and then later report back on the therapeutic success or failure of the treatments you have tried out.

ABOVE *Grill the therapist before starting treatment.*

THE "BACK SCHOOL"

As the term implies, a "back school" takes an educational approach. Back pain sufferers attend classes where they are taught about the anatomy and physiology of the spine, what to do, and what not to do. Sessions may also involve group exercises for the back, and possibly an element of counseling.

This approach often works very well. Thorough reviews of the subject imply that back schools are most effective when intensive sessions are held in the workplace. It also makes sense, of course, to combine attendance at a back school with a comprehensive treatment plan. Understanding your own back is clearly a good thing. If nothing else, it helps to prevent you from panicking about back pain, and stops bad postural habits.

BELOW *Students keep their own file of notes.*

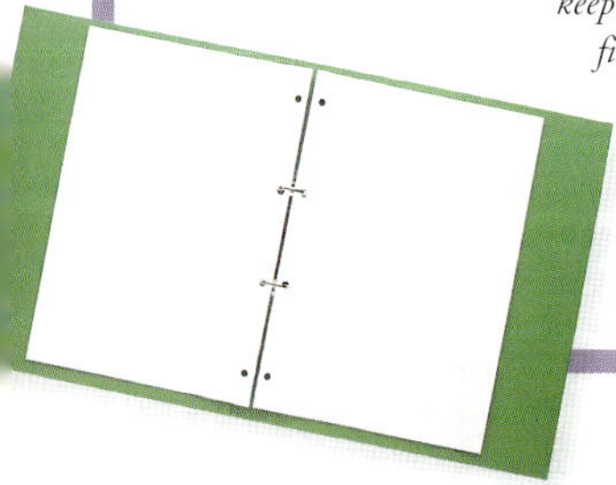

BACK LESSONS

Instructors teach techniques to use for everyday activities. Sharing experiences with others in the class may also be helpful. The exercises learned may prevent recurrence of backache.

DOES IT WORK?

Research results on back schools are not uniform, but many trials suggest that they successfully prevent back problems. In one study, for instance, it was shown that after attending a back school, bus drivers were on average about 20 percent less affected by back pain in the following year.

BACK LESSONS

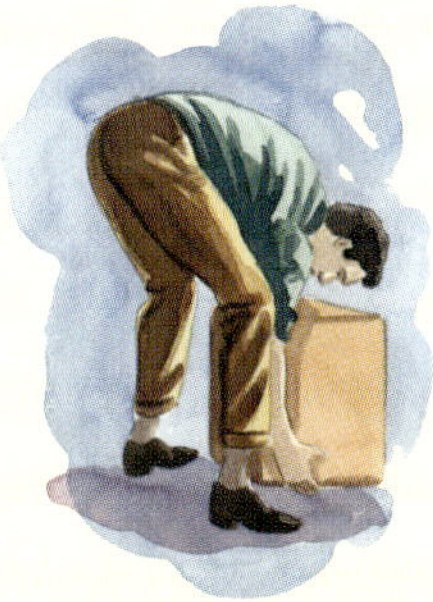

INCORRECT

Do not bend over from the waist to lift: this puts maximum stress on the spine. Bend your knees, and lift the weight from a crouched position.

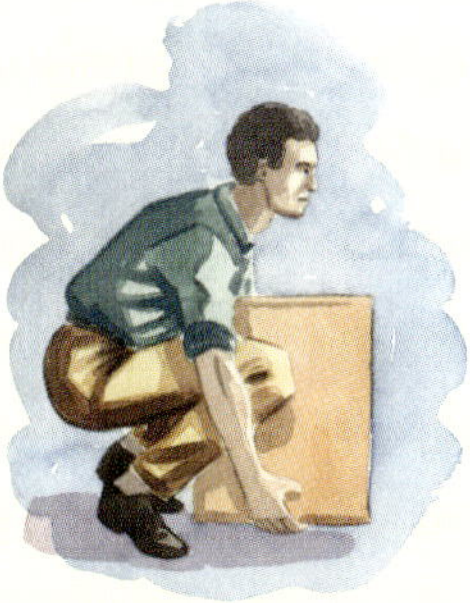

CORRECT

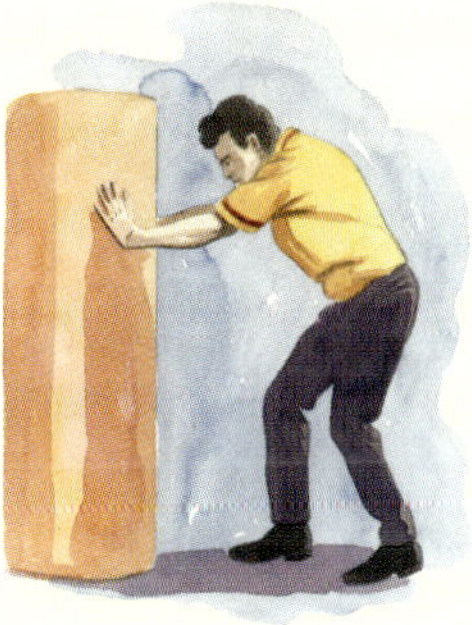

INCORRECT

Do not stand away from a heavy object you are trying to move. Instead, lean against it and "put your back into it" by pushing from the floor.

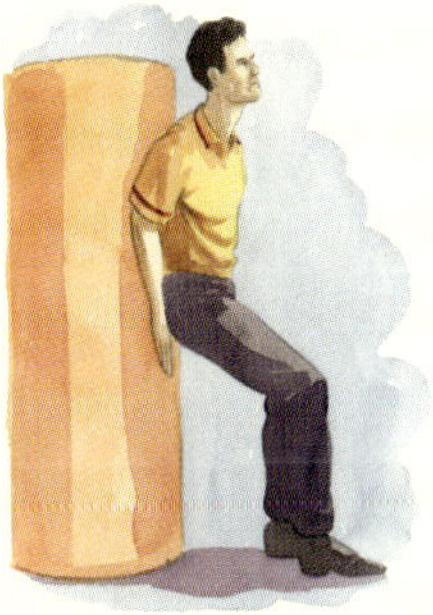

CORRECT

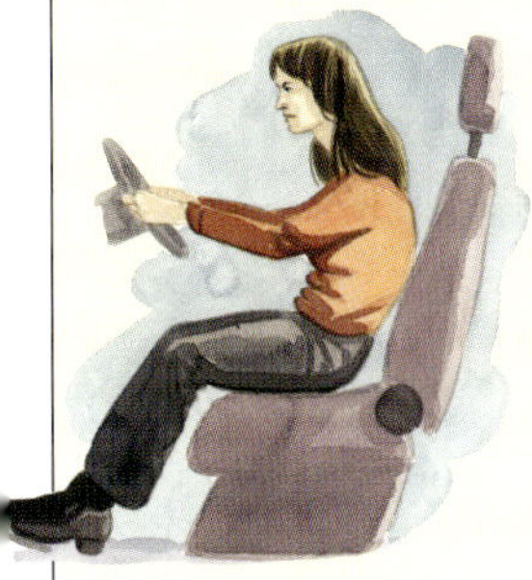

INCORRECT

Do not drive in a slouched or hunched position. Make sure the spine is well supported, in an upright position. Avoid long drives.

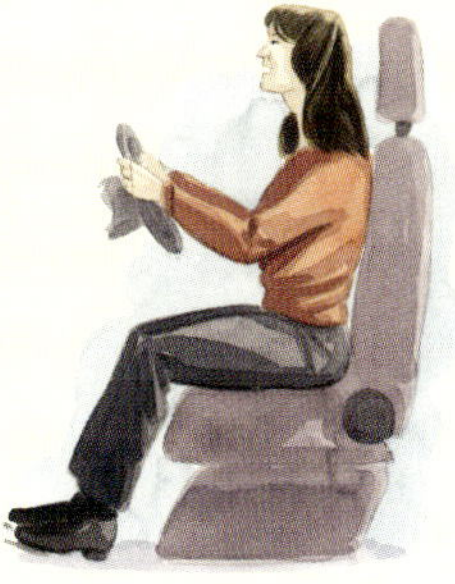

CORRECT

PREVENTING BACK PAIN

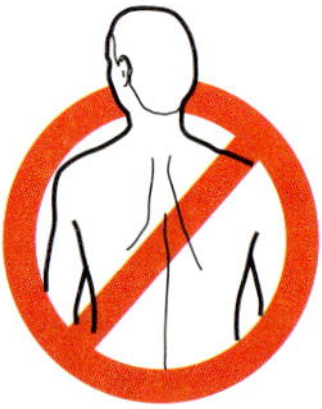

ABOVE *Be aware of potential back dangers.*

Back pain is so widespread that almost all of us do, or will, suffer from it – it's virtually an epidemic. Epidemics are best confronted not by treatment, but by prevention. It makes a lot of sense to apply this principle to back pain.

If we accept that treating back pain is not always successful, then maybe the best approach is to prevent it from occurring in the first place.

THE RISK FACTOR CONCEPT

Most diseases are not the result of a single cause, but the complex interaction of a multitude of risk factors. It is worth knowing about these contributory risk factors for at least a couple of reasons.

REDUCING THE RISK FACTOR

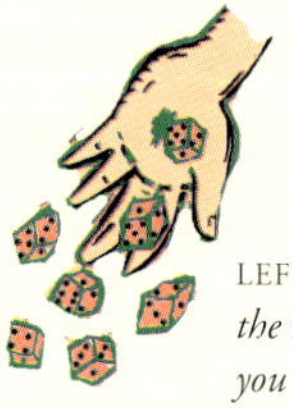

LEFT *Know the risk factors you run.*

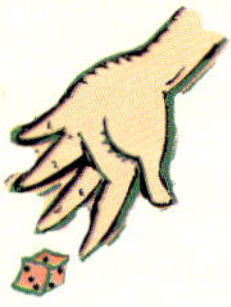

RIGHT *Reduce those that you are able to.*

• If we can change or eliminate a risk factor (e.g. smoking), we reduce the risk. This means we decrease the probability that we will be affected by back pain.

• If we cannot do much about a risk factor (e.g. body height), we still profit from knowing about it. We would know, for instance, who is at a particularly high risk and therefore has to take other preventative measures particularly seriously.

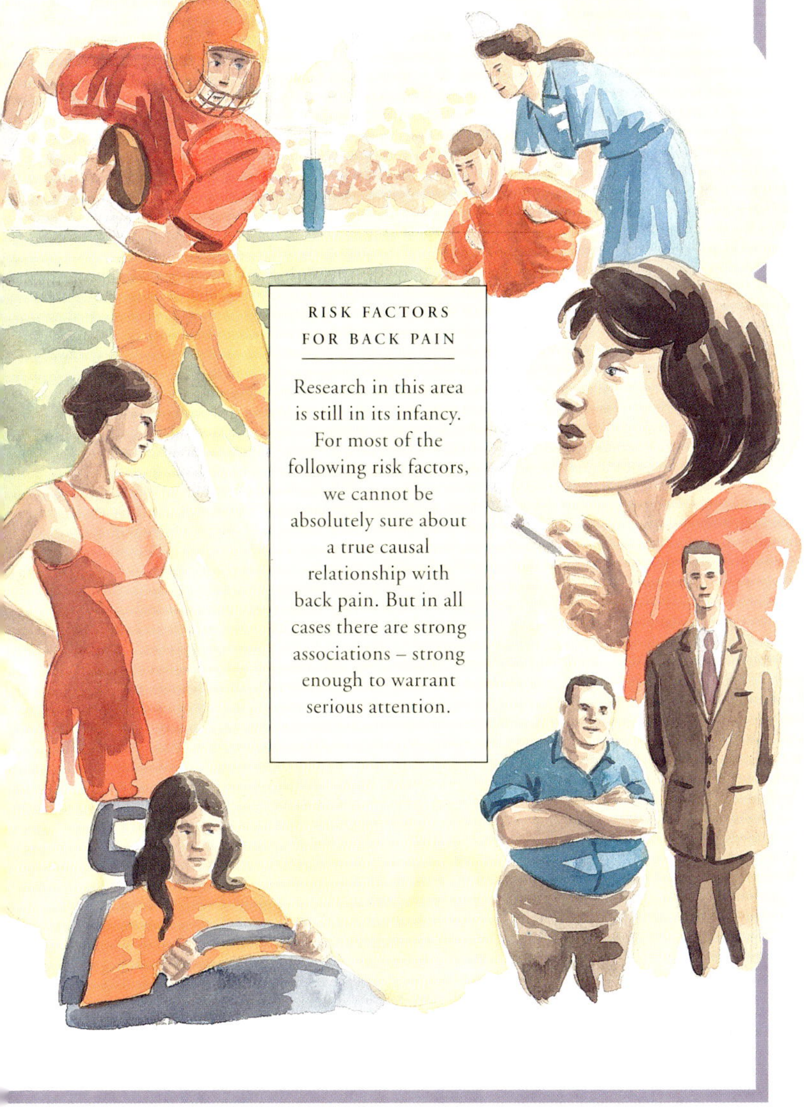

RISK FACTORS FOR BACK PAIN

Research in this area is still in its infancy. For most of the following risk factors, we cannot be absolutely sure about a true causal relationship with back pain. But in all cases there are strong associations – strong enough to warrant serious attention.

PHYSICAL ACTIVITY

In a way, exercise is very much a two-sided coin. On the one hand, exercise strengthens the back and trunk muscles. This in turn stabilizes the back and prevents back problems. On the other hand, we know that certain movements and activities put an extremely high strain on the back, which can obviously cause injury to the back and pain.

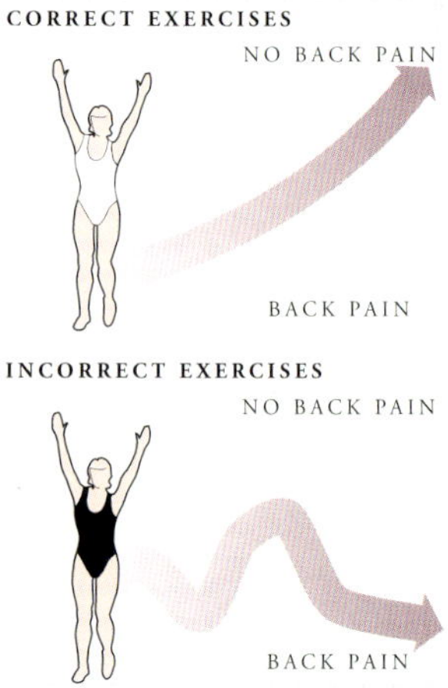

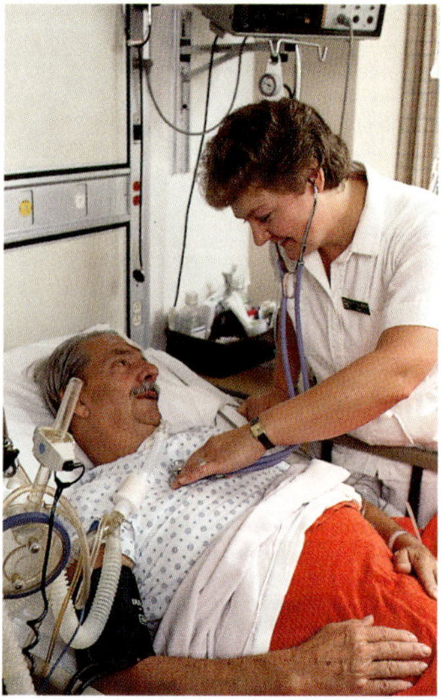

ABOVE *Nurses must be wary of the cumulative effects of lifting patients.*

Research has shown that individuals who are well trained and have strong trunk and back muscles, are less likely to suffer from back pain than those who are less well trained. Once you have had an episode of back pain, you can also reduce the likelihood of it recurring by taking up exercises that strengthen the muscles along your back and, just as importantly, those on your stomach.

There is also ample evidence to show that certain physical tasks, particularly when carried out every day at work, lead to back problems. Several professions have been cited as particularly vulnerable.

- ***Miners, often working in bent positions.***
- ***Nurses, often lifting heavy loads.***
- ***Workers in the car industry, often lifting in a bent position.***
- ***Packers, often rotating the spine under load.***

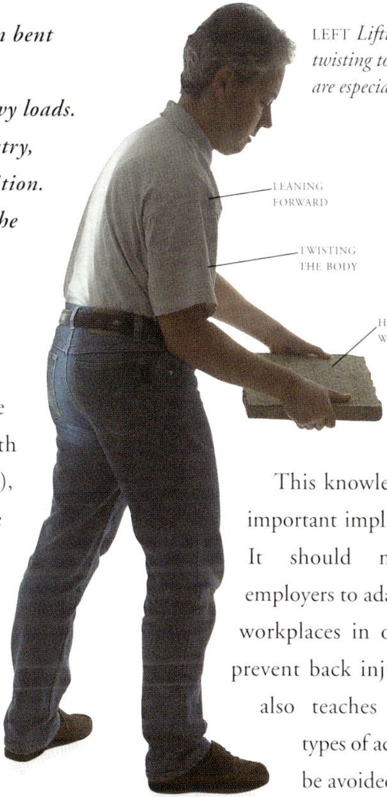

LEFT *Lifting and twisting together are especially bad.*

A common theme emerges from looking at these professions: workers make repetitive movements with additional load (as in lifting), in positions where the spine is bent forwards, and this is particularly harmful. The danger of back injury is even higher if rotational movements are carried out under these conditions.

This knowledge has important implications. It should motivate employers to adapt their workplaces in order to prevent back injuries. It also teaches us the types of activity to be avoided.

EXERCISES TO STRENGTHEN THE BACK

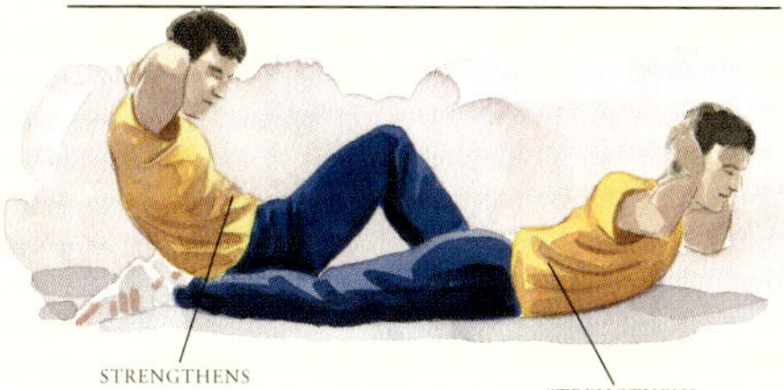

RIGHT *Sit-ups strengthen abdominal muscles as well as back muscles.*

LEFT *Keeping the hips on the floor, lift the head and upper body.*

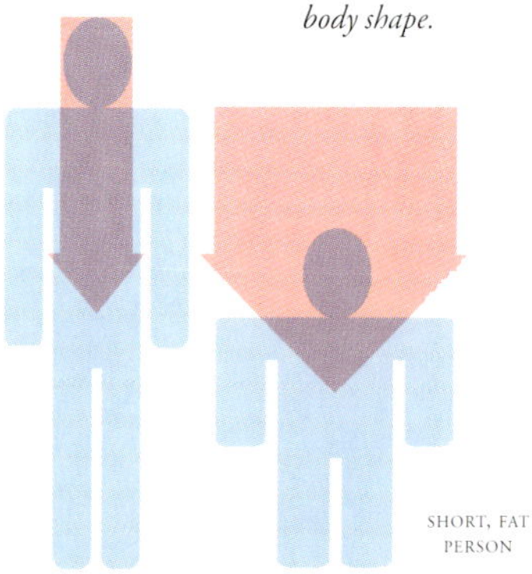

BELOW *Risk factors concurrent with body shape.*

BODY HEIGHT AND WEIGHT

It follows that the more stress and strain we put on our back, the more prone to problems it will be. It is logical that tall people (through the height of the spinal column) put more pressure on their lumbar spine than short people. A heavy person puts more pressure on the spine than a thin one. Research has confirmed that obese people have about a 50 percent greater chance of suffering from back pain. For body height, the situation is similar. Tall people are two to three times more likely to end up with recurrent back pain.

The implications are clear. You can't very well shorten your body height but you can (and should) lose weight if you are overweight. This may alleviate back problems and help to prevent their occurrence.

THE SITTING POSITION

Many of us work in professions where we remain in postures that are not natural for humans, and which put mechanical stress on our spine. Often this will be the sitting position. While sitting, the strain on the lumbar spine has been measured to be extremely high. There are, however, good and bad sitting positions. We should take great care that our office furniture is adapted to our needs.

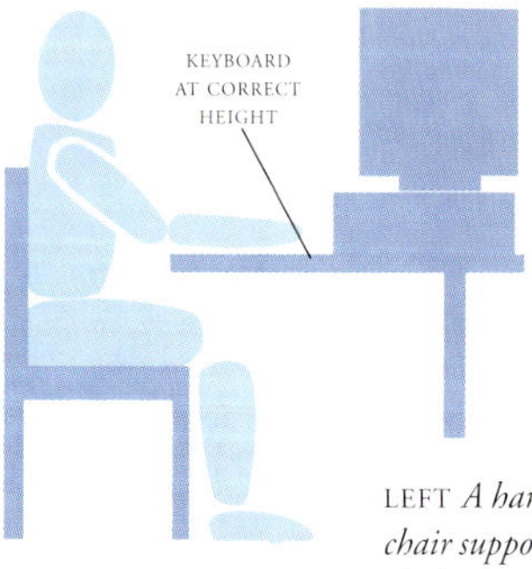

LEFT *A hard chair supports the back.*

The issue is of obvious and particular importance for our children. Schools still rarely take much notice of the importance of correct sitting posture. Classrooms should be equipped with the right seats, taking into account the variation in body size that may exist within one age group. Teachers should learn the essentials of correct sitting and see that this knowledge is applied in their classes.

DRIVING A CAR

When driving a car, we are not always seated in the optimal position. Often we can't move or change position for a long time. We have our arms stretched out, which puts additional strain on the back. And we are submitted to continuous vibrations from the car which are suspected of having detrimental effects on the back. All these factors add up, rendering driving a particular risk for back pain.

Research has shown that the chance of suffering from back problems increases with the time spent driving a car. Professional drivers are twice as likely to have back pain as other people. The comfort of a car seat is important: people using well-designed car seats suffer only about half the problems of those using an uncomfortable car seat.

The message here is clear: choose your car seat carefully. You can't tell a good seat from a bad one by just looking at it or sitting in it for a minute or so. Test drive a car extensively before you buy it.

CAR SEAT CHECKLIST

Some important features of car seats are:

✧ Lumbar support.

✧ Armrest.

✧ Support on both sides of the torso.

✧ Headrest.

✧ Extensive adaptability of the sitting position.

✧ Non-slip seat covers.

BELOW *Look for a good, supportive car seat.*

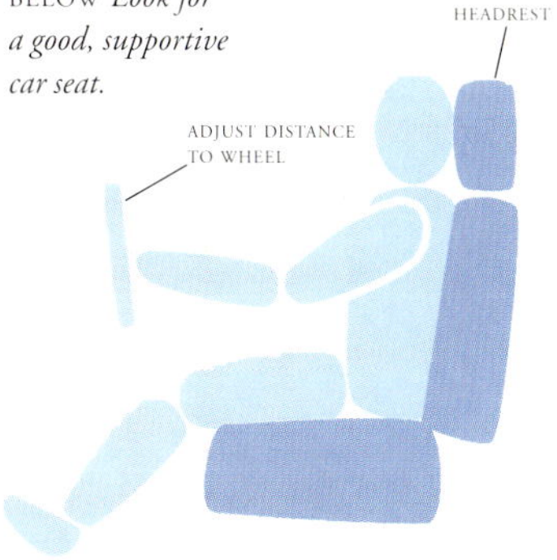

FAMILIAL PREDISPOSITION

Of course, we can't exchange our parents, but it is very important to know whether back pain runs in families. The subject is complex, but there is some evidence to suggest that such a predisposition does, in fact, exist. For instance, if you suffer from back pain, there is a 35 percent chance that a close family member does also.

There also seems to be a genetic predisposition that increases the risk of back pain for Caucasians by about 40 percent over that of other races. Men also suffer slightly more often than women – but this, as we have seen, could have to do with their larger weight and height.

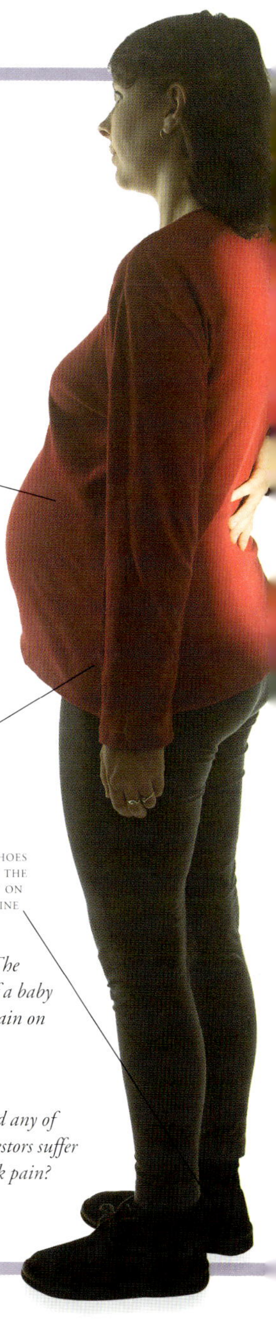

RIGHT *The weight of a baby puts a strain on the back.*

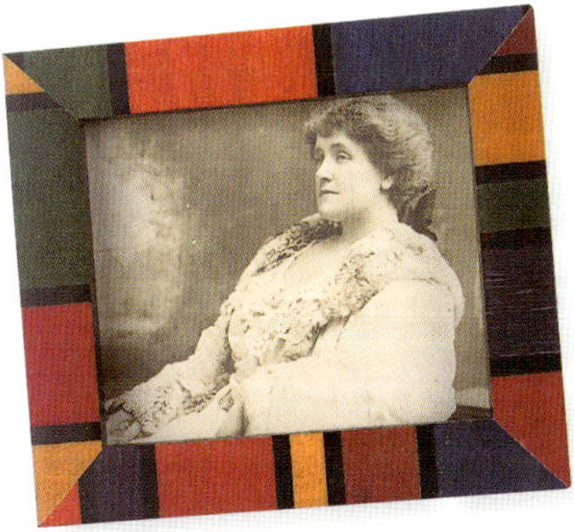

LEFT *Did any of your ancestors suffer from back pain?*

PREGNANCY AND THE CONTRACEPTIVE PILL

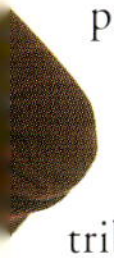

We know that pregnant women frequently suffer from back pain. This probably has several causes. The mechanical strain of the additional weight could be a contributing factor. Also, during pregnancy, the female body produces a hormone called relaxin. It helps relax the ligaments and enables the pelvis to expand and harbor the growing fetus. But it also relaxes the ligaments in other parts of the body, such as around the spine. Thus the spine becomes more vulnerable to injury and more prone to back pain.

What has back pain got to do with taking the contraceptive pill? The answer is simple: recent research has shown that the pill has similar effects on relaxin levels to a pregnancy. Research from Scandinavia suggests that this makes the pill a risk factor for back pain. One should, however, stress that these are preliminary results and that the issue is complex. If these findings are confirmed, they imply that stopping the pill is a preventative measure against back pain.

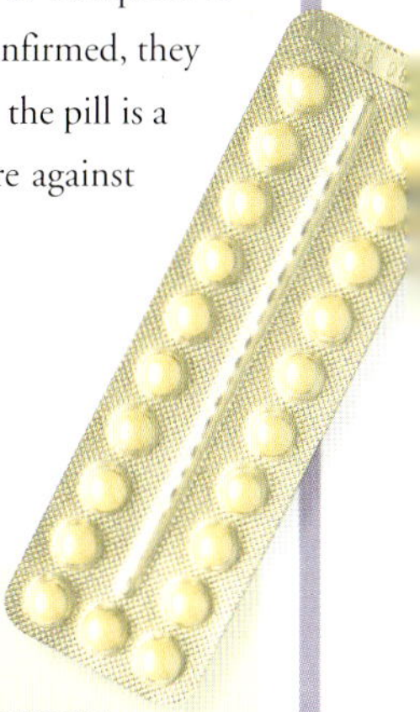

RIGHT *Contraceptives are suspected of being a risk factor.*

RELAXIN LEVELS

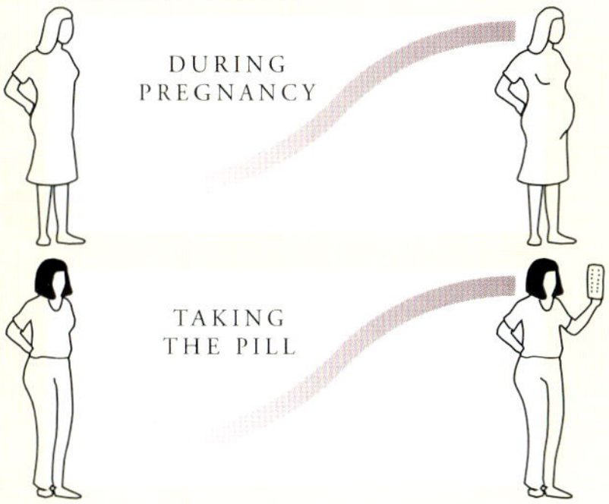

The body produces a hormone called relaxin during pregnancy to relax ligaments in order to accommodate the growing fetus. The contraceptive pill also causes relaxin levels to rise in a similar fashion, relaxing ligaments and rendering the spine more prone to pain and injury.

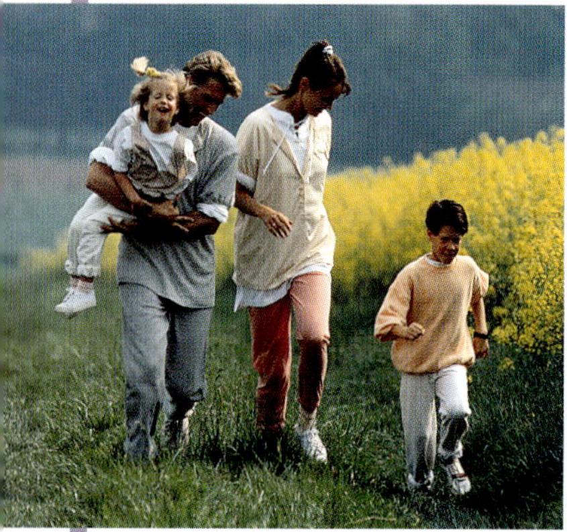

ABOVE *Protect your children from passive smoking.*

SMOKING

Smoking is a prominent risk factor for circulatory disease and cancer, and it may also be a risk factor for back pain.

This may come as a surprise to most people, but it is not as implausible as you may think. In fact, the mechanisms by which smoking causes heart attacks and back pain may be quite similar. Smoking seriously limits blood supply in any tissue of the body. In the heart this can lead to a heart attack, in the brain to a stroke, and in

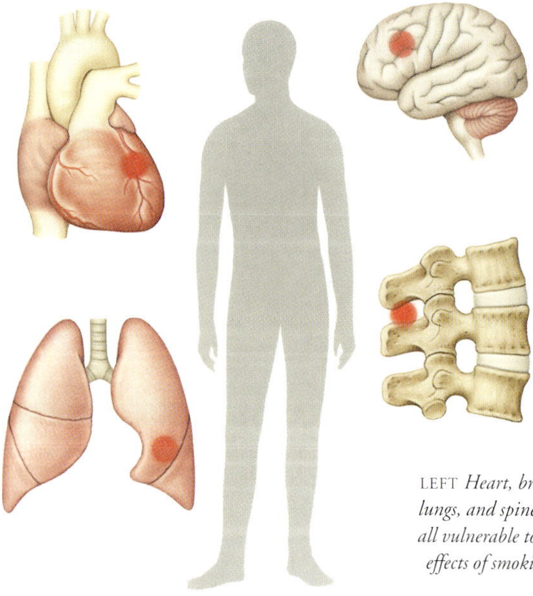

LEFT *Heart, brain, lungs, and spine are all vulnerable to the effects of smoking.*

the back to pain. Poor blood supply to the various tissues around the back means that they become more prone to injury, and that the body's natural ability to repair damage is impeded. The bottom line is that back pain may result.

SMOKE ALARM

Heavy smokers are about twice as likely to suffer from backache as non-smokers.

RESEARCH

What does research tell us? Most studies on the subject implicate smoking. One US investigation found that heavy smokers were about twice as likely to suffer from backache as non-smokers. Others found a fairly clear-cut relationship: the more you smoke, the greater the risk of ending up with a back pain problem. Scandinavian researchers recently tackled the problem in a different but revealing way. They observed a large group of smokers for thirteen years. Those who were affected by back pain had a five-fold increased risk of dying from heart disease. Collectively, these and other research findings make it likely that a link does exist between smoking and back pain.

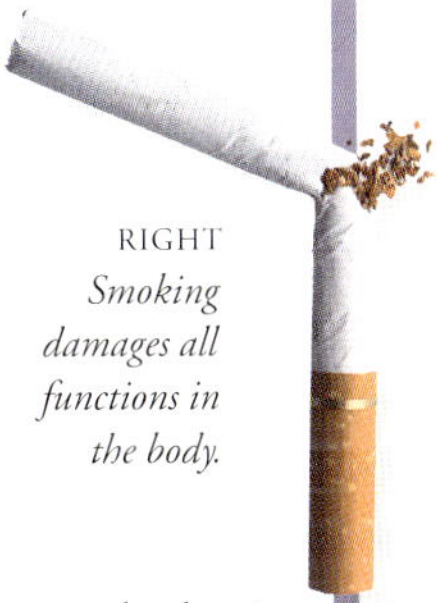

RIGHT *Smoking damages all functions in the body.*

If you are a smoker and want to prevent back pain from developing in the future, do your best to give up the habit now. You'll also benefit from a lessened risk of acquiring various other diseases.

ISK OF BACK PAIN

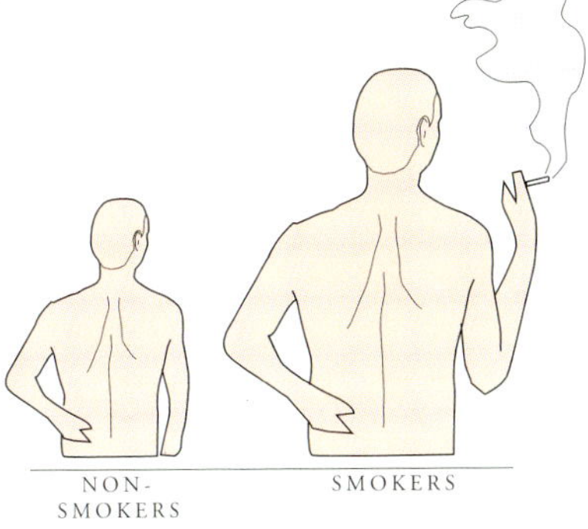

LEFT *Smokers run the risk of increasing their chances of suffering from back pain.*

HOW CAN COMPLEMENTARY MEDICINE HELP PREVENT BACK PAIN?

Complementary medicine can contribute to the prevention of back pain in several ways. Whether you have chosen spinal manipulation, yoga, the Alexander Technique, or other complementary options, most therapists will teach you about correct body posture and remind you how to move without hurting your back.

LOOKING AT THE WHOLE LIFESTYLE PICTURE

Good complementary practitioners have a holistic outlook, and will try to see your problem in the context of your entire life situation and advise you accordingly. They will discuss healthy eating, your optimal body weight, the importance of regular activity and following a healthy lifestyle. Such advice may help to eliminate the risk factors, boost general health, and reduce the likelihood of back pain or its recurrence.

A HOLISTIC APPROACH

Holistic medicine believes that ill-health is caused by an imbalance of all the facets of a person's life, and that in order to treat illness, lifestyle should be examined. The whole person is treated, to enable the body to heal itself.

Think about the compartments of your everyday life, the people you interact with, your work and leisure time. How do these things affect your general well-being?

- Your spiritual life: happiness and satisfaction levels, moods, emotions, and temperament.
- Your relationships with others: family and friends, colleagues, general social life.
- Your work: is it satisfying and productive, or are you constantly stressed and overworked?
- Your diet: is it healthy and rich in nutrients, or do you exist on snacks, rushed meals, and junk foods?
- Your leisure time: do you make the space in your life for real relaxation by taking a break from everyday routine, and following your hobbies?
- Your exercise schedule: do you try to fit some form of regular exercise into your life?

SPIRIT
Pay heed to your emotions and feelings, and try to achieve inner harmony.

RELATIONSHIPS
Put energy into improving relationships with family, friends, and colleagues.

EXERCISE
Exercise three times a week for twenty minutes.

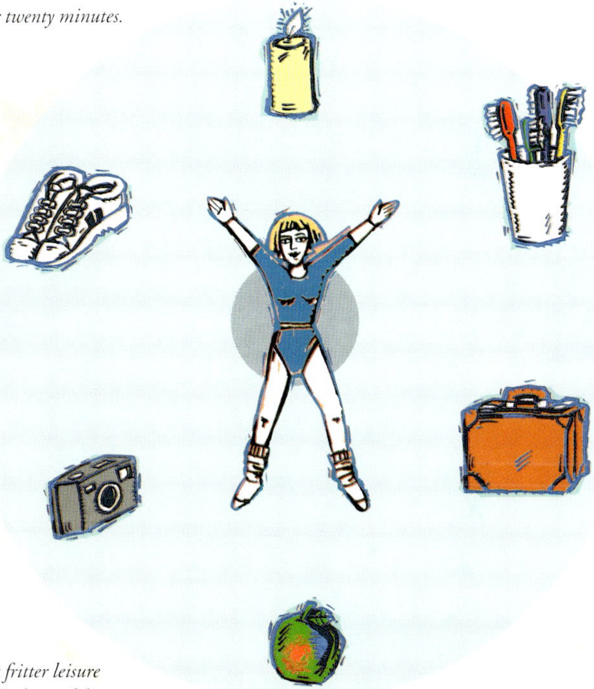

FUN
Don't fritter leisure time in front of the TV: do something more productive.

FOOD
Choose foods wisely, but don't deny yourself an occasional treat.

WORK
Try and take a balanced approach to work and don't let things get on top of you.

BACK PAIN AND SPORT

Some sports are good for the back, in that they may help to prevent recurrences once an episode of back pain has subsided. Others put a lot of strain on the spine, and may therefore lead to back problems.

It is therefore important to differentiate carefully between sports that benefit and those that harm your back. If you currently suffer from backache, you should certainly not overdo any physical activity. Wait until the pain is bearable; subsequently you may take up a sensible leisure activity. But do take it easy! It is important that you enjoy exercise – so choose a sport to try out that you really fancy.

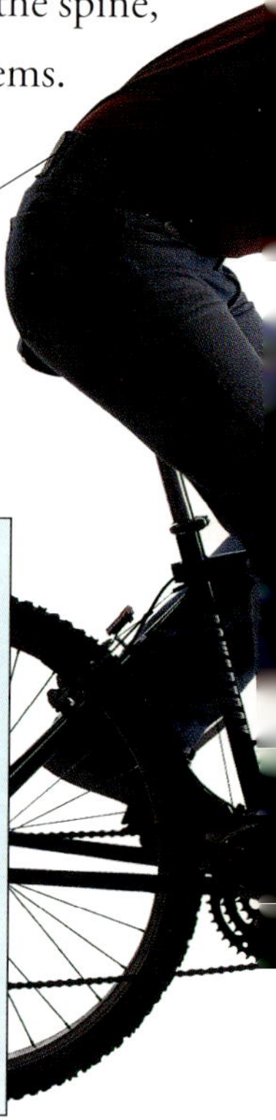

SPORTS THAT ARE KIND TO BACKS

The types of sport that are normally good for your back include:

- ✧ Cycling
- ✧ Riding
- ✧ Swimming
- ✧ Walking or moderate running

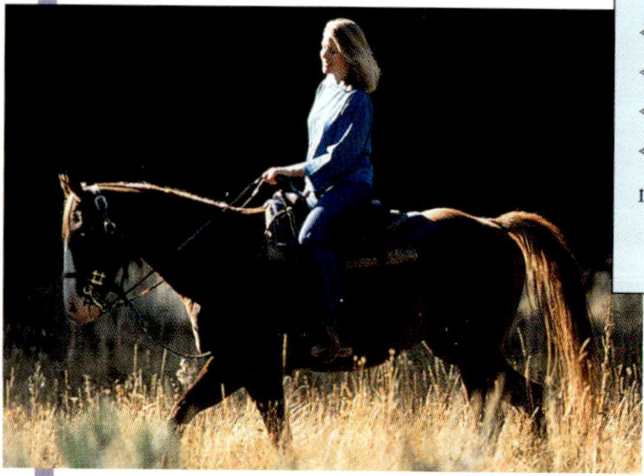

LEFT *Riding is suitable for people prone to back problems.*

BELOW *Cycling is an easily accessible sport – just set off!*

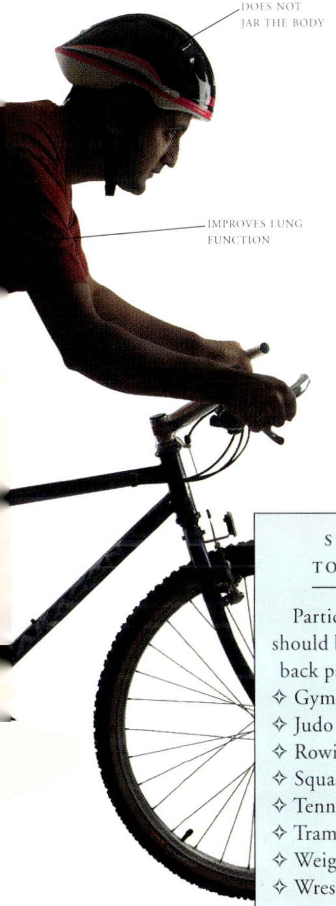

DISC DANGER

The intervertebral disks are mechanically highly vulnerable *(see pages 14–19)*. Their low metabolic rate prevents them from keeping pace with the adaptive processes that happen throughout our life. Therefore abrupt increases in physical activity, particularly at later stages in life when we are unaccustomed to heavy physical load, can easily injure a disk and cause back problems. Any unusual strain to the back is dangerous. If you are not accustomed to a sport, for instance if you were once active but have not trained for years, make sure that you take it easy. Start with very low-intensity training; increase exercises slowly as your body re-adapts to the unfamiliar strain.

High-risk activities for backs are those which engage only one side of your back, such as tennis, those which put a lot of weight on it (weightlifting), and extreme movements (gymnastics).

SPORTS TO AVOID

Particular sports should be avoided by back pain sufferers:

- Gymnastics
- Judo
- Rowing
- Squash
- Tennis
- Trampolining
- Weightlifting
- Wrestling

PRACTICAL TIPS FOR BACK PAIN SUFFERERS

Control your posture whenever you can (e.g. when sitting at your desk or driving)

✧

Remain active even during an episode of back pain. Return to work as soon as you possibly can

✧

Avoid repetitive lifting and carrying heavy loads Use the correct technique when lifting is unavoidable

✧

Avoid twisting your back, particularly when carrying a heavy weight

✧

When carrying a load is unavoidable, distribute it evenly (e.g. rucksack on both shoulders)

✧

Sleep on a good orthopedic bed and mattress

✧

Use the correct technique for getting up

✧

Use a good, adaptable chair in the office

✧

Make sure your car seat suits your back

✧

Avoid long periods of time in one posture (e.g. sitting)

✧

Avoid awkward postures as much as you can

✧

Avoid long car journeys

✧

If you have to drive a long distance, make sure that you take regular breaks, possibly including simple exercises for your back

✧

Avoid frequent bending forward

✧

Get physically fit through progressively increasing regular exercise

✧

Do exercises, particularly when your back pain has gone

✧

Avoid whole body vibration (e.g. machinery)

✧

Avoid mental stress

✧

Avoid a too-fast work pace

✧

Avoid monotonous work where you can

✧

Try to achieve work satisfaction as much as possible

✧

Do not consent to repeated X-rays without good reason

✧

Avoid prolonged bed rest even when you have back pain

A COMPREHENSIVE TREATMENT PLAN

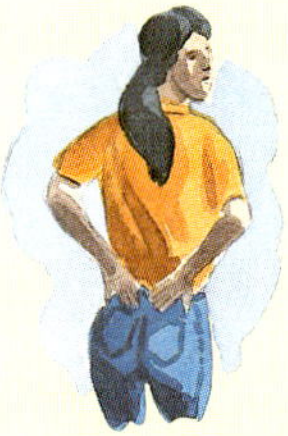

ABOVE *You may feel pessimistic about recovery to begin with.*

REMEMBER

1. Back pain is not a distinct disease entity but a symptom. This means that one back pain is not necessarily like another back pain.

2. There can be no "golden rules" and each treatment plan has to be highly individualized. It must take into account:

- ***The nature of your particular back problem.***
- ***Your signs and symptoms.***
- ***Your entire life situation, worries and hopes.***
- ***Your previous experiences with certain forms of treatment.***
- ***The prognosis for your condition.***
- ***The possibility of preventing further episodes of back pain.***

AIMS

To get you symptom-free as soon as possible and to keep you out of trouble in the future.

STRATEGY

A comprehensive plan will often need more than one therapeutic approach. Educating yourself, together with a combination of conventional and complementary treatments, is the best strategy. Once the pain has gone, put the emphasis on prevention of further back pain episodes.

FINALLY

The most important thing about treating your back pain is to remain as active as you can and to regard the problem not as a disease, but as a normal event that affects us all.

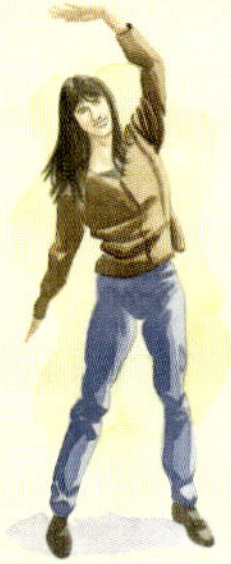

ABOVE *But remember you will soon regain full mobility.*

FURTHER READING

SUITABLE FOR LAY PEOPLE

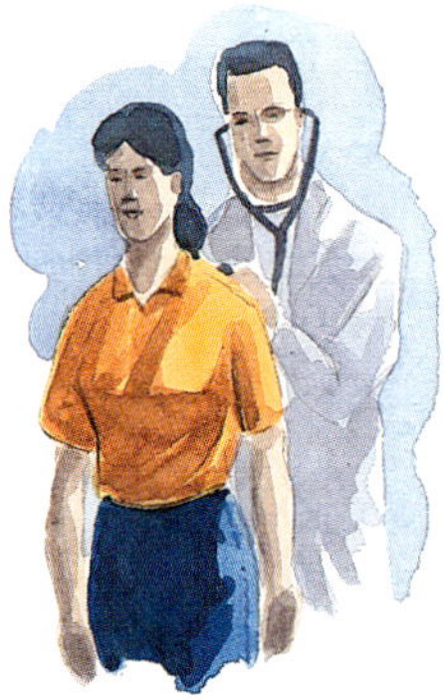

Cassileth, B.R.
The Alternative Medicine Handbook
(Norton WW, US, 1998.)

Fugh-Berman, A.
Alternative Medicine: What Works
(Odonian Press, US, 1996.)

Ernst, E. (ed.)
The Book Of Symptoms And Treatments
(Element, UK, 1998.)

Jayson, M.I.V.
Back Pain, The Facts
(Oxford University Press, UK, 1992.)

Maxwell-Hudson, C.
The Complete Book Of Massage
(Dorling Kindersley, UK, 1988.)

The Back Book
(Published in the UK by HMSO. ISBN 00117020788.)

Understanding Acute Low Back Problems. A Patient Guide
(Published in the US by Dept. Health and Human Services. AHCPR Publ. No. 95-0644.)

Vickers, A.
Massage And Aromatherapy
(Chapman Hall, UK, 1996.)

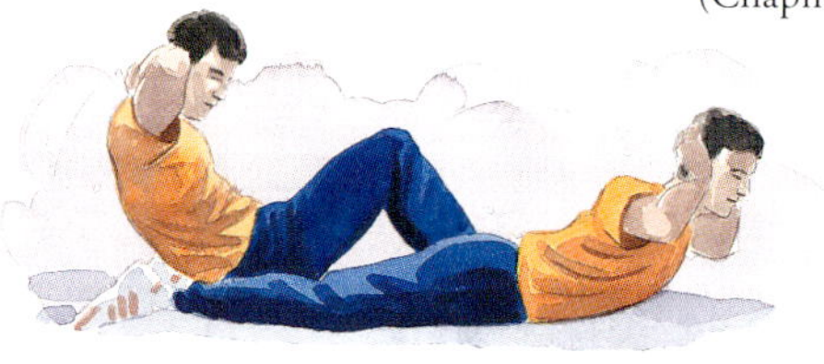

MORE SUITABLE FOR PROFESSIONALS

Baldry, P.E.
Acupuncture, Trigger Points And Musculoskeletal Pain
(Churchill Livingstone, UK, 1993.)

Bensoussan, A., and Myers, S.P.
Towards A Safer Choice
(Southern Cross University, Australia, 1996.)

BMA
Complementary Medicine: New Approaches To Good Practice
(Oxford University Press, UK, 1993.)

Ernst, E. (ed.)
Complementary Medicine: An Objective Appraisal
(Butterworth, UK, 1996.)

Ernst, E., and Hahn, E. (eds)
Homeopathy: A Critical Appraisal
(Butterworth Heinemann, UK, 1998.)

Filshie, J., and White, A.R. (eds)
Medical Acupuncture: A Western Scientific Approach
(Churchill Livingstone, UK, 1998.)

Giles, L.G.T., and Singer, K.P.
Clinical Anatomy And Management Of Low Back Pain
(Butterworth Heinemann, UK, 1997.)

Huang, K. Ch.
Acupuncture. The Past and the Present
(Vantage Press, US, 1997.)

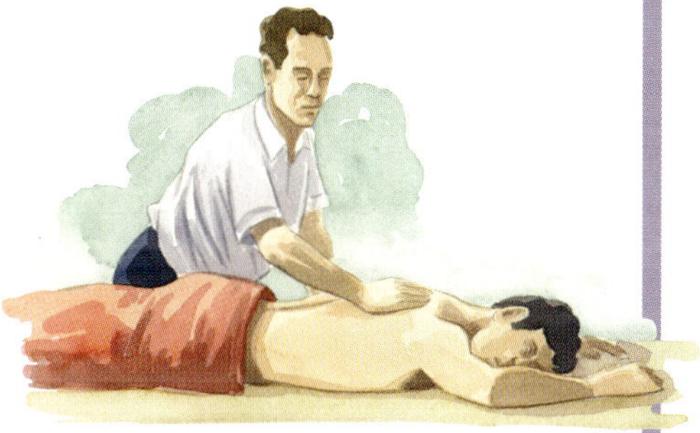

Murtagh, J., and Kenna, C.
Back Pain And Spinal Manipulation
(Butterworth Heinemann, UK, 1997.)

Wirth, S.
Integrative Medicine
(Creative Logic, US, 1998.)